SAVING JACK

Saving

A Man's Struggle
with Breast Cancer

Jack

JACK WILLIS

Foreword by
Alan B. Hollingsworth, M.D.

UNIVERSITY OF OKLAHOMA PRESS: NORMAN

Library of Congress Cataloging-in-Publication Data

Willis, Jack, 1940–
    Saving Jack : a man's struggle with breast cancer / Jack
Willis ; foreword by Alan B. Hollingsworth.
        p.   cm.
    Includes bibliographical references and index.
    ISBN 978-0-8061-3895-4 (hardcover : alk. paper)
    1. Willis, Jack, 1940—Health.   2. Breast—Cancer—
Patients—Oklahoma—Biography.   3. Cancer in men.
I. Title.
    RC280.B8W472 2008
    362.196'994490092—dc22
    [B]   2007024203

The paper in this book meets the guidelines for permanence
and durability of the Committee on Production Guidelines
for Book Longevity of the Council on Library Resources. ∞

1 2 3 4 5 6 7 8 9 10

CONTENTS

FOREWORD

Alan B. Hollingsworth, M.D.

　　　　　　　　　　　　*

Seven centuries have passed since an English surgeon, John of Arderne, first described breast cancer in a male. Remarkably, history scrolled through its pages for the next seven hundred years without a book on the subject. So, when journalism professor Jack Willis first felt a lump beneath his nipple, page one of a new tale began.

Sure, there are pamphlets that cover bare-bones facts about male breast cancer, plus random tidbits online. A page or two will appear in the medical books on cancer as well. Yet, even breast disease texts pay scarce attention to the subject. In one of the thickest references, boasting 1,631 pages overall, only five pages are devoted to male breast cancer. Until now, no male breast cancer patient has tackled the shock of being diagnosed with "a woman's disease" through a book-length chronicle of the experience.

Men usually have well-honed methods to deal with stress, techniques that go by a variety of sophisticated terms, though "stuffing" covers it pretty well. Authors, however, have learned to deal openly with the causes of such stress. So, it makes sense that it took the occurrence of breast cancer in a male journalist to prompt the writing of this premier book.

What the reader will encounter here goes far beyond an antiseptic account of prickly needles and eager scalpels. While the hard-nosed realities of facing cancer therapy are vividly described, what is most intriguing in *Saving Jack* is the backdrop story of one man forced to contemplate the big round period that punctuates the end of life.

No one coasts into middle age without experiencing some trauma. Fortunately, most of us become adept at stowing away these memories and, though not forgotten, nor particularly in peace, they rest in waiting. Then, when our health is threatened to the point we concede we are just mortals, these life-shaping tribulations have a way of coming on deck once again. This is the intrigue of *Saving Jack*.

Peeling away one layer at a time, the author reveals stories that few of us will experience, while other themes are common to all. We are all different, all the same. In *Saving Jack*, both the foreign and the familiar are brought home through the author's skillful weaving of the tough times arising from his cancer diagnosis along with examination of the relationships that have defined his life.

Few men will travel this same road. Only two thousand men per year in the United States will hear these words: "You have breast cancer." Some 450 men per year, diagnosed previously, will hear even worse: "Your breast cancer has spread." The natural history and treatment are remarkably similar to the disease as it occurs in women, though one of its peculiarities is the greater likelihood of the tumor being influenced by the hormone estrogen. Most men are prescribed the very same anti-estrogen drugs given to women to treat breast cancer. And while the textbooks dwell on the risk factors associated with male breast cancer, just as we have long lists of risks for females, most men in the United States with the disease have none of these identifiable risks. It just happens, and future generations of researchers will eventually figure out why.

When women are diagnosed with breast cancer, they face issues of body image and sexuality that cannot be completely understood by men. Yet, as soon as a woman learns of her diagnosis, she has the potential to be enveloped by old and new friends who have already had the same experience. In most locations, support is available for those who seek it—women sharing with women exactly how they coped with the problems unspoken in mixed company.

But when a man is diagnosed with breast cancer, he will be hard pressed to find another like soul. And while he doesn't suffer the same impact from disfigurement (though some men undergo reconstructive surgery), there is a trade-off. Facing the same risk of death as a woman with breast cancer, the man will find no structured support system in place. Some male breast cancer patients try to blend into the female support systems, where sometimes they are accepted with enthusiasm, but sometimes not. For some women, the loss of a breast supersedes the brush with death, and they rebuff their male counterparts who have undergone mastectomy: "After all, what did he really lose?"

Where does a man with breast cancer turn? In *Saving Jack*, the breast cancer patient turns to family and friends. Family and friends do not need to be affected by breast cancer to pour out love and empathy. Thus, the basis of a true "support group" is not necessarily the sharing of the same disease. Rather, it's the communal effort of surrounding a loved one with outstretched arms and saying, "You may teeter back and forth during this tribulation, but we're here to catch you if you start to fall."

Value every page of this book, for if history repeats itself, we might be waiting another seven hundred years for the next tome to cover the experience of what it's like to be a man diagnosed with a cancer thought to be reserved for the opposite sex.

PREFACE

I turned over in bed and looked at the digital clock on the night table. The red numbers glowed in the dark. I squinted and tried to focus. It was 3:30 A.M., and I couldn't go back to sleep.

I wasn't feeling the effects of the chemotherapy or the drug-induced nightmares or the dry mouth. I wasn't feeling depressed or lonely or scared. Actually, I felt just the opposite: optimistic, inspired, and energized.

I'd just had a brainstorm, a why-didn't-I-think-of-this-before inspiration. I decided to write a book. I wanted to wake up Becky, my wife, and tell her my revelation. On second thought, my timing might be off. I'd wait until she woke up to tell her.

I'd never written a book, but I was a journalist. It couldn't be that difficult, could it? Never mind that the longest article I had ever written was a sixty-inch newspaper story. Never mind that I didn't know the difference between a preface and an afterword. That didn't matter. I wanted to tell other newly diagnosed cancer victims, their families, and their friends some of the things our family didn't know about cancer when I was diagnosed.

First thing when we crawled out of bed, I told Becky. She liked the idea—a survival story about a man with breast cancer, stereotypically a woman's disease. The concept for book was born.

Saving Jack is about my struggle—my family's struggle—with cancer. It's about how the disease affected me as well as Becky and Stephanie, our married daughter. It's about handling emotion, some of which is linked to gender. It's about challenges and adversity and triumph.

Our story is about some of the simplest things in life, things we take for granted, and things we never expect to lose. It's about walking the dog and planting tulips—the trivialities of life, the small pleasures that can occupy a day and make it complete. It's about some of the most important things in life too, those things we may not give enough attention to. It's about love and family and prayer, and the fear that I could be seeing the azaleas of spring and the sunflowers of summer for the last time.

Our story is about having a support system and the graciousness to accept help when it's offered. When Becky would ask someone other than myself for help, it used to bother me. Before we married, I dropped by her house to help fix an electrical problem in the bathroom. It chafed me a bit when I saw Frank, Becky's dad, up on a ladder helping her. It didn't matter to me that I knew absolutely nothing about electricity, nor did it matter to me that Frank was a retired electrician.

A couple of years ago, Becky wanted our son-in-law, Chap, to replace a faulty faucet in the kitchen. I asked why she needed his help. I would do it. For some reason, I never got around to it. We paid Home Depot an arm and a leg to replace the faucet.

I was diagnosed with invasive ductal carcinoma in February 2005 and experienced a mastectomy, chemotherapy, and radiation treatments through September of that year. The cancer dramatically changed my life's routine. The way I went about my day, the way I looked at life, the way I thought. This ordeal, this disruption, has been most difficult, and the aftereffects remain to this day. Edginess and irritability rear their ugly heads more often, but I see what's important—and sometimes it isn't what I thought it was.

ACKNOWLEDGMENTS

How do you thank someone for saving your life? *Saving Jack* is about those people who helped me battle breast cancer. My eternal gratitude goes to my family and friends, my co-workers and students at the University of Oklahoma, and my doctors and nurses.

First, I thank my wife, Becky, and our daughter, Stephanie. They contributed to this book, a story incomplete without their perspectives. More important to me is their support and love. I thought I had the world by the tail when Becky and twelve-year-old Stephanie agreed to marry me. Little did I realize the depth of love, the warmth, and the life fulfillment that awaited me. Stephanie brought her husband, Chap, into her life and into our family. Chap loved and comforted her and made her stronger during this cancer crisis.

I am indebted to . . .

Becky's sisters, Gigi and Francie; my late brother and sister-in-law, J.B. and Charlotte; and our extended families, who supported and prayed for us.

Judi, for looking out for Becky and giving her a time-out every so often, and for being her friend.

Bill and Patti, for all of the support, friendship, and advice they gave us.

Debbie and Jim, for giving Becky a job that allowed her time to take care of me.

Ilene and Ann, and Kathryn and Ryan, for the caring and thoughtfulness of good neighbors.

Twila, for giving me friendship, advice, and the daily inspiration and motivation to continue my work.

My students, who were my pillars. They made each day a little easier. Many trusted me enough to share their own personal tragedies and problems in dealing with cancer, either their own or their mother's or their father's. I didn't name students in this book, not because I didn't truly appreciate them, but because I didn't want to take advantage of their status for my own purposes.

My former students who came to the OU Relay for Life from Dallas, Tulsa, Oklahoma City, Muskogee, and Washington, D.C., and other alumni who supported me from Portland, New York City, St. Louis, and Austin, Texas, and a hundred other places.

My coworkers and friends Susan, Clarke, Nancy, Allison, Stacy, and Michael, for being there, for wearing those yellow bracelets of support, and for brightening the days when I didn't feel well.

Karen and Nancy, both oncology nurses and breast cancer survivors; Dr. Tom Shi Connally, general surgeon; Dr. Stephen Lindsey, family physician; Dr. Sherri S. Durica, medical oncologist; Dr. Glenda K. Young, radiologist; and Dr. Robert Gaston, radiation oncologist.

A special thanks to Lori Brooks, who performed a first edit on the manuscript; Kathryn Jenson White, an OU journalism professor who encouraged me and provided ideas for this book; and Jim Davis, an OU professional writing professor who encouraged me and provided advice for publishing.

And finally, to my editors at the University of Oklahoma Press whose suggestions made this book so much better and who made my first attempt into book publishing such a joy: Charles E. Rankin, associate director and editor-in-chief, and Alice Stanton, special projects editor.

SAVING JACK

1
THE DISCOVERY

I was in the shower when I felt a pea-size nodule under my right nipple. It startled me. I had never felt any lumps on my body, except for the occasional calcium deposit and the time my childhood friend Billy Mutzig hit me in the head with a chunk of wood.

This lump was small, though. Probably nothing to worry about. I'm a guy, right? Still, I slid my finger over it again and slowly circled it. It felt rubbery and seemed to move when I crowded it. I soaped again and went on with my business.

I usually think about other things while in the shower. I don't pay much attention to scratches and bruises, except after a day of reckless weed eating and lawn mowing. Those battle scrapes smart. This lump was different, though, and in a different place; no weed-eating welt there. I wondered.

The blurry image of my wife, Becky, flashed past the fogged glass door of the shower. I stuck my head out from under the spray, pushed open the door, and flagged her down.

"Can men get breast cancer?" I asked.

Becky, my wife of twenty years, and I had gone through what we thought was a rough year in 2004. We lost her father in February, my sister in March, and my former brother-in-law in April— too much grief for one year.

I had become close to Frank, Becky's dad, over the years. I grieved more for him than I did when my own father died a decade earlier. I knew Frank didn't have long to live, but I wasn't prepared for the loss. I suppose nobody ever is.

My sister's death left only three siblings from my family of nine. I was the youngest. My mom and dad, three sisters, and a brother were gone. You pay a price for being the baby. You go through the pain of losing everybody—one by one, heartache by heartache.

My former brother-in-law had become like a big brother to me during the twenty years of my first marriage. Though we hadn't spent time together lately, I still felt the love and the loss when he died.

Things happen in threes, my superstitious nature told me. Three deaths. Three months. Surely, nothing else would happen, I thought. I was wrong.

In May, Abby, our dog, broke Becky's fingers. Abby was a one-hundred-pound border collie mutt, and Becky was a one-hundred-pound petite redhead. Becky had the leash wrapped around her left hand when Abby lunged at another dog. The force crushed Becky's hand, breaking the middle two fingers in thirteen places. Surgeons operated on her fingers in June.

Afterward, Becky developed a chronic pain disorder—reflex sympathetic dystrophy, or RSD—and went through seven months of physical therapy. She regained about 70 percent mobility in her left hand but still had pain.

I took out my frustration on the dog. I was so angry with her that I tried to give her away, but I couldn't find any takers. Who wanted a big ole mutt anyway? I thought about returning her to Second Chance, the animal shelter. But after I simmered down, I remembered how pitiful—and how lovable—she was when we found her there as a four-month-old pup. All of her eight brothers and sisters had found new homes. All but her. She was the last of the litter, and nobody wanted her. I couldn't take her back.

Becky and I gave up plans to return to Branson, the country-music resort near the corner of southwest Missouri and northwest Arkansas, where we usually vacationed in May and August. By fall, we were looking forward to a better year in 2005.

Becky and I led the simple life. We put Paris Hilton and Nicole Richie to shame when it came to simplicity. Our little world was on the plains of the heartland, fifteen miles from Oklahoma City. We had migrated from the hills and lakes of eastern Oklahoma to Norman a decade earlier. We were Okies from Muskogee and proud of it.

I was a newspaper editor for twenty years before becoming an instructor at the University of Oklahoma and advising the student newspaper, *The Oklahoma Daily*. Becky, as a vice president, managed loan departments at two banks and at two savings and loan institutions during the 1970s and 1980s, the bank scandal years. She worked for federal regulators in the early 1990s when they started closing banks nationwide. She swore she knew where the Clinton Whitewater skeletons were buried.

When we moved to Norman, she didn't want to work for a bank again. She wanted to sell clothes. I'd never seen a woman who loved clothes as much as she did. Imagine a 25 percent discount off a pantsuit already marked down 75 percent; Becky called it heaven. She worked for Dillard's department stores in Norman for nine years, selling petite women's clothes and serving as a consultant for Liz Claiborne.

We had an active lifestyle. I walked three miles at 6 o'clock most mornings, and Becky and I had begun to hit tennis balls again before the dog broke her fingers. We gardened, frequently walked the neighborhood together, and worked out three or four times a week. When we vacationed in Branson, we traipsed up and down the hills on the six-mile strip and spent hours wandering through the outlet malls. I didn't smoke or drink. I considered myself somewhat fit, if not entirely firm.

As each year slipped by, we fought harder to avoid the golden years. We thought about what we would do after I quit work. (In 2003, I had checked to see what my pension would be if I retired at sixty-five. I quickly determined I would have to work the rest of my life—or starve to death.) We had talked with Stephanie, our thirty-something daughter, about downsizing and what we would like to do when I eventually retired. We had considered living on the same property—building a big house for her and her husband, Chap, and a small house for us. Even though it was all talk, I had begun to think seriously about the winter of my life. And not just about money.

I worried because Becky smoked. I wasn't concerned about secondhand smoke. I was thinking of her health. She would try to quit time and again without success. She would quit for a week or a month; then a crisis would happen, and she would light up.

If she wasn't addicted to nicotine, she was obsessed with her looks. Every time she tried to quit, she gained weight and stressed out. She smoked when she was nervous, not because she enjoyed cigarettes. When she quit smoking, she ate to curb her anxiety. She tried the patch, cessation classes, gum, cold turkey. Nothing seemed to work.

She knew about lung cancer. Her mom, a smoker, had died of lung cancer in 1997 at age seventy-two. Her dad, a smoker, had died at eighty-two in 2004, but he didn't have cancer.

Why do people do something they know can be detrimental to their health? Why do they regularly eat too much? Why do they refuse to exercise? Why do women fail to get mammograms? I don't know.

Becky called our friends Dr. Bill Shelton and his wife, Patti, and asked them to go to dinner with us. We ate Mexican food, and then Dr. Bill chauffeured us back to our house to see the new sunroom, still unfinished, and drink orange smoothies.

The four of us made small talk and relaxed before Becky asked Dr. Bill if he would take a look at my little nodule. He put on his doctor's face, that serious demeanor I had seen before in the emergency room.

"Can I take a look?" he asked.

I began to get nervous. I pulled up my shirt and Dr. Bill's fingers examined my right breast. I was familiar with his work from my kidney stone adventures in the Norman Regional Hospital emergency room.

Dr. Bill was a good physician, and I trusted his opinion. I sometimes wondered if he and other doctors and lawyers ever questioned a friendship when their friends asked for professional advice. My editor instincts told me they did. I should have asked him if my impositions offended him.

Becky and Patti had met when Patti was shopping at Dillard's. They became friends, and that relationship branched out to include Dr. Bill and me. Dr. Bill was laid-back. I was laid-back. Patti was spunky. Becky was spunky. The four of us hit it off right away.

Dr. Bill recommended I have a biopsy performed. I made an appointment with my family doctor, Stephen Lindsey. He felt the lump, and then checked for enlarged lymph nodes around my neck and under my arms. He asked if the nodule hurt or bothered me. It didn't. He agreed with Dr. Bill. I needed a biopsy. He referred me that day to a general surgeon.

The surgeon examined both my breasts and the lymph nodes around my neck and shoulders. His fingers dwelled on the mysterious little mass just below my right nipple. I fidgeted, but the lump didn't hurt and I didn't mind the examination. He asked if I had any tingling in my extremities, any shortness of breath, any pain anywhere, and if anyone in my family had cancer. My sister, who had recently died of Parkinson's disease at age seventy-three, had had cancer, but it had been in remission for years.

My lump was soft and mobile, the surgeon said, and cancer is hard and fixed. He said he was 99 percent sure the nodule was not malignant. He said he wasn't worried and told me to come back if the nodule grew.

"If you're not worried," I said, "then I'm not worried."

Over the next few weeks, I pretty much stopped thinking about the little mass. Actually, I felt very comfortable not thinking about it. Dr. Lindsey recommended that I not feel it unnecessarily, so I didn't. Every couple of weeks, though, I brushed the soap a little slower across my right breast. The nodule didn't get any bigger, and I had more serious problems to worry about at the time.

Probate proceedings for my late sister's estate in Tennessee had become a quagmire of delays and complexities by December. The Nashville court had appointed me administrator of the estate. I was waiting out a four-month public-notice requirement before I could close out her affairs. On the date I expected a favorable ruling, the judge balked at a routine request for an accountant's fee. He wanted a detailed written statement to support the claim.

As a former newspaper editor, I had learned not to get too upset when things didn't go my way, but I also knew a thing or two about judges and the court system. I was hot. I stayed up until 4 A.M. researching computer files and paper records for the past eight years and preparing a five-page letter to the court. I learned a lesson that night: Put your estate in a trust so you don't have to probate it.

I was still angry as I slipped into bed. When I woke up two hours later, I couldn't stand up. Every time I tried, I got dizzy and lay back down on the bed. I felt nauseous.

"My God," I thought. I might be having a heart attack or a stroke. (Sometimes I thought I was a hypochondriac.)

Becky thought I should go to the emergency room. She took my blood pressure every five minutes for the next half hour.

Instead of sending me to the ER, Dr. Lindsey agreed to see me that morning. Where else in America can you get a doctor's appointment the same day you call in? He diagnosed the cause of my problem as not eating well for a couple of days, staying up late the night before, and being stressed by the probate ordeal.

Since I was already in his office, I asked him to check out the nodule again. I thought it had grown. Dr. Lindsey thought so too. He said that once the probate was settled, the nodule needed to be taken out.

I felt tired at times during the late fall, and I told Becky I guessed I was just getting old. I was sixty-four, but I had always acted and felt younger than my age.

Through the fall, I had a periodic itching in my right nipple, the one close to the lump. When I scratched the nipple, the sensation was soothing. It felt like scratching poison ivy initially, before the scratching becomes painful. I never scratched long enough to see if it would hurt. The left nipple never itched, and I wasn't smart enough to ask the doctor about it. I guess I thought I was experiencing some sort of aphrodisiac the boys on the playground never told me about.

My moment of reckoning with the mysterious little mass came on Monday, February 7, 2005. I was in the shower. I brushed the soap across my right breast, and I felt something. I stopped washing abruptly. Water drenched my head and shoulders and ran down my body. I stood paralyzed in a warm basin of water.

The tumor was frighteningly larger than the last time I felt it—as much as five times larger. Once I summoned the courage to touch it again, the area around it felt squishy and spread out like a ganglion cyst that had been smashed. I panicked and stopped feeling it. The mass had inched lower, almost down on my rib cage, rather than up close to the nipple where I'd first noticed it.

The moment I felt the mass, I knew it was cancer. I hoped it wasn't, but I knew it was. I felt petrified. You know the feeling—that flushed, fuzzy sensation that starts in your head, swirls around, and streams down through your chest, your arms, your stomach, and your legs to your toes. That out-of-control instant when you're slipping on ice and you're going down. You're helpless, and a sick-to-your-stomach feeling engulfs you. If I ever had a moment during this entire ordeal that I realized cancer kills and I could die, that was it.

The day I discovered the tumor had mushroomed, the day my life speed-shifted into high gear, I called to set up another appointment with the surgeon. The receptionist said he had retired from surgery on January 1. First, he said he was 99 percent sure my lump wasn't cancer. Now he was retired. Just great! The receptionist said the doctor still practiced, though, and could take a look the next day. Okay, then.

Becky and I waited anxiously in the examination room, fearing the diagnosis. The doctor remembered me. He smiled and said it had been a while. I noted the irony. I slipped off my shirt and scooted up on the cold examination table. He gently moved his fingers around the area below my right breast. His probing made me uneasy this time, unlike in June. It didn't hurt, but it bothered me. The doctor didn't say a word. Then he examined my left breast and the lymph nodes under my arms. Since he no longer performed surgery, he referred me to a new surgeon in town.

The receptionist told me the new doctor, Dr. Tom Shi Connally, was the nephew of my boss's wife, Molly Shi Boren. My boss was David L. Boren, the former Oklahoma governor and U.S. senator who was now president of the University of Oklahoma. I thought the family connection might get me a discount. It didn't.

Dr. Connally examined me. He said he needed a biopsy of the tumor because it was so big and had grown so fast. That was the only way to determine if it was malignant.

"Cancer or not, it's got to come out," he said.

I lay on the examination table, getting chilled and wondering when he would schedule the biopsy and surgery. My teacher's thought process kicked in. How was I going to work this into my class schedule, into the newspaper's schedule? I couldn't just up and leave work for my own convenience.

If I had to have surgery, I thought spring break, six weeks away, would be the best time. If surgery were early that week, I could get on my feet before students returned from their vacation. Becky and I could get the yard in shape. We had plenty of work to do before I could consider surgery. Six weeks sounded about right. I expected doctors could fit surgery into that time frame. The life-and-death nature of cancer had escaped me for the moment.

Dr. Connally laid out a plan that changed my life quickly and forever:

- I would have a biopsy procedure in the hospital's Breast Care Center the next day. (The nurse made arrangements with the hospital as we spoke.)
- I should call the hospital myself and schedule preoperative testing.
- The following Monday, Dr. Connally would see me in his office.
- In one week, on February 15, 2005, I would go into surgery for either a lumpectomy or a mastectomy, depending on the biopsy results.
- Dr. Connally would be the primary surgeon.
- Any questions?

I looked at the doctor and then at Becky. I needed a minute.

2
THE BIOPSY

I worked at school the next day before Becky and I went to the hospital for pre-op testing and an ultrasound-guided biopsy. Pre-op testing included a vitals check, a finger prick for a blood sample, an EKG, and a chest X-ray. As I lay on my back with heart-machine tentacles draped over my chest, the ceiling fascinated me. A collage of man's best friends stared down at me. Color pictures of cute puppies, ugly puppies, bulldogs, mama dogs, and every other kind of canine imaginable entertained me while the machine did its work.

The testing completed, we crossed the corridor to the Breast Care Center for the biopsy. A nurse escorted me to an examination table. While she moved my table around and readied a monitoring device, she explained the biopsy process. Christian music from a CD player wafted through the room.

The nurse asked what kind of music I liked. I said, "Enya." She inserted a different CD, and the haunting strains of Enya's "Only Time" began to play. Is that a great hospital or what?

Another nurse, Karen Saunkeah, applied the local anesthesia—a series of injections, in a cluster much like the pattern of a tuberculosis shot—around the area of the tumor. Karen said she was a breast cancer survivor herself. I began to pay more attention to what she was saying. She'd had a mastectomy a few years earlier. In her four years at the hospital, she had seen only two men with breast cancer. I knew I was special.

A burning sensation stung my chest as she administered the needle pricks to deaden the area. She told me the radiologist would use a piece of equipment that sounded very loud when the needle was injected.

When the local anesthesia had done its work, the radiologist demonstrated the needle gun. She squeezed off a test round so I could hear the bang. It sounded like a staple gun—a loud whack.

A cell phone rang. The doctor, two nurses, and Becky all reached for their cells. It was Becky's. A student reporter needed me. Becky told the reporter I would call back; then she turned off the phone.

The radiologist held the gun against my skin and fired—whack—sending a needle spiraling into the tumor. The needle collected its evidence—a core sample of tissue—and retracted. I felt the gun's pressure against my side; it was uncomfortable but not painful. Enya had long since faded away. I focused totally on what this person with the gun was going to do next.

She fired a second spear, this time from a different angle. I experienced more pressure, but still no pain. Becky said my legs were as rigid as a board, and my feet and ankles were crossed and locked. Not the picture of relaxation. As if she knew what was coming—mental telepathy, I suppose—she stood up from her chair and grabbed hold of my legs.

The doctor fired a third round. Whack!

Whoa! My shoulders tensed, and my body bucked like I had been shot. The needle missed the deadened area and streaked across my chest. Wow, that smarted. It felt like a tiny bullet piercing my chest muscles. The searing sensation lasted no more than fifteen to twenty seconds, but it seemed longer.

The doctor apologized and said she needed one more sample. I cringed and watched her stick the gun to my side. Whack! A clean shot. I relaxed.

Nurse Karen said the doctor would call around 2 or 3 o'clock the next day with the biopsy results.

As Becky drove me back to work, a million thoughts darted through my mind. What will the biopsy show? Maybe the tumor is benign. What does cancer feel like? What if I have more tumors? If it's malignant, what will happen to me? What if the cancer has spread? What will happen to my family? How will this affect my job? Can I still work? I can't afford not to work. How much does cancer cost?

Will insurance pay for everything? What if it doesn't? What if they didn't catch it in time?

If it is cancer, how far has it progressed? I kept mulling one question over and over in my mind: What if they haven't caught it in time?

Becky drove me back to work. We rode silently, with our thoughts consuming us. I assumed Becky was thinking the same things. She thought of something more.

"I'm going to be pissed if it's cancer," she blurted out.

I looked at her quizzically and then began to laugh, the kind of laughter that releases tension and makes everything seem all right. She laughed, too, at the double meaning of her outburst. It was clear, though, that she had not forgotten what the first surgeon had said back in June. He'd been 99 percent sure the pea-size nodule wasn't cancer. Neither of us had ever thought I would be in that other 1 percent.

I married Becky after knowing her for three months.

Her telephone voice intrigued me when I called her the first time. A mutual friend had set us up on a blind date for lunch. I picked up the two of them, and we went for Chinese. Shortly after I got back to the office, I called to ask Becky for a second date. Her phone voice mesmerized me. It was deep and sultry and hot.

On our second date, we ate dinner at the all-you-can-eat buffet at Fin and Feather Resort on

Lake Tenkiller. I didn't realize until later that Becky didn't like all-you-can-eat buffets. She was petite and couldn't eat that much. The banker in her thought it was a waste of money to pay for food you didn't eat.

Aside from taking her to the wrong restaurant, I stuck my foot in my mouth on the way back to Muskogee. I told her I had gone out with a couple of women since I had been widowed.

"One was divorced."

"Really," Becky said. "I've been divorced twice."

Oops.

"Oh, not that I minded," I said. "I was just mentioning it. There's nothing wrong with being divorced."

Becky laughed at me.

"Do you go to church?" I asked. She probably thought I was giving her the third degree.

"Yes. First Methodist."

"First Methodist? That's where I go."

"No, you don't," she said. "I've never seen you there."

"I'm an usher."

"Really? I work with the youth at Sunday school. Sometimes I don't go to the church service. When we do, Stephanie and I sit down front on the right side, usually with my sister and our friends."

"That explains it," I said. "I work the back left side. I sit back there."

How strange that was. I couldn't believe I had never seen her. The congregation wasn't that big, but I didn't go to Sunday school. And I suppose if a person wasn't looking for a romantic relationship, he might not notice a beautiful woman. What kind of guy doesn't notice a beautiful woman?

For a while, Becky had worked three jobs to support herself, and Stephanie, a twelve-year-old latchkey kid at the time. They ate peanut butter sandwiches for breakfast, lunch, and dinner.

Becky had a strong type A personality. I liked spirited women, and it didn't take long to figure out I'd found one. She was a pistol. She had a fiery temper and liked her space.

"I'm very independent," she said, as soon as we started dating. Setting the ground rules, I assumed. "I've never accepted help from anyone."

She told me she had given up on men.

"No offense. All the good ones are taken," she said. "I just decided to put my life into Stephanie, church, and work."

"No offense taken."

I was forty-four. I knew what I wanted in a woman: integrity, genuineness, charm, spirit, courage, wit, fiscal conservative, liberal philosophy, beauty, warmth, passion, a Christian. I knew I had found those qualities—all of them—and I fell for her.

We set out on a whirlwind romance. We each had a mental checklist of what we wanted in a partner. When we compared lists, we found we were a match. We clicked.

I knew she was the one I wanted. I was afraid that if I asked her to marry me, though, she would turn me down. I hated rejection. I didn't know how to propose. Sitting on the couch in her living room one night in October 1985, I simply blurted it out.

"What would you say if I asked you to marry me?"

"Are you asking?"

"What would you say if I was?"

"I'd say yes."

"Well, then I'm asking. Will you marry me?"

"Yes," she said, without a moment's hesitation. "But would you rather just live in sin?"

I thought she was kidding. She wasn't.

"Absolutely not," I said.

She mentioned one more ground rule.

"I've dealt with everything myself and I always like to be in charge of the finances, the entertaining, things like that," she said.

"Hmmm. She wants to wear the pants," I thought.

I was accustomed to taking care of my own finances. I had to think about that—for about two seconds. Here was a banker. Who was more conservative with money than a banker? And she was a vice president. The bank obviously trusted her.

Agreed.

There was just one more matter to settle: the twelve-year-old, a pistol in her own right. I knew a lot of stepfathers and stepchildren had problems. But I quickly became enamored of Stephanie. She answered the door the first time I picked up Becky for a date.

Stephanie seemed so grown up. She didn't look like a grown-up, but she acted like one. Her looks, bobbed haircut, and cheerful demeanor made me think of a pixie. Four foot six. Seventy-five pounds. Strawberry blond hair. Blue eyes. And when she smiled, her eyes twinkled. Her face lit up, revealing braces, top and bottom, and big dimples.

What impressed—and surprised—me most were her manners, confidence, and poise. Her personality was bubbly, enthusiastic, and, I suspected, mischievous. I didn't know how a preteen was supposed to act, but I thought this one was way beyond her years. She was the perfect hostess.

"Hi. I'm Stephanie," she said, flashing a wide grin. "Mom's not ready yet. Won't you please come in?"

She escorted me into the living room, offered me a seat on the sofa, and excused herself. I overheard bits and pieces of her conversation with her mother.

"Mom, he brought chocolates!"

"What's he wearing?" Becky asked. "I don't know what to wear."

The first month we dated, Becky asked me if I would like to go with Stephanie and her to Wal-Mart. Not your typical date. What couple goes to Wal-Mart when they've just met? But I had managed a five-and-dime store for ten years before I went to work for the newspaper. I liked retailing. I wanted to go with them. I didn't know it at the time, but Stephanie had thrown a fit with her mother because she didn't want me tagging along.

"We girls didn't need you around," she told me years later. "Did you have to go everywhere Mom and I went?" She apologized for that tantrum. She said she didn't realize when Becky married me that her mom was giving her a father.

After Becky and I decided to get married, we talked with Stephanie. I desperately wanted her approval.

"Stephanie, I've asked your mother to marry me. Will you marry me too?"

Her eyes widened, and she flashed that big grin.

"Yes," she said.

Stephanie and I never had a problem. As the years passed, she gave me all I could have ever hoped for. She told me she wished I were her real father. To me, she was always my daughter, not my stepdaughter. Stephanie got a kick out of it when we introduced each other as father and daughter, and people would say, "I see the resemblance."

"You let me know when I was wrong, and lifted me up when I was right," she said later. "You let me talk about how I felt when Me-maw died and no one else would listen." She remembered my being there for her dance recitals, cheerleading tryouts, football games, driving lessons, broken hearts.

Stephanie played second base on the middle-school softball team and guard on the basketball team and was a cheerleader. As a high school sophomore, she tried out for the cheerleading team. She had even taught one of the senior girls, who had never been a cheerleader, how to cheer. The senior made the team. Stephanie didn't. I cried more than she did that day.

Steph and I were a lot alike. Our birthdays were in October, seventeen days apart. She and I laughed at the same corny jokes and cried over the least little thing. But then, she was still her mother's daughter: sensitive and nurturing, yet strong, fearless, and assertive. She stood up for what she believed was right. She could take care of herself.

Becky and I set a June wedding date but quickly changed our minds. Why wait? We weren't kids. We knew what we wanted. We married in January 1986.

3
IT'S CANCER

By midmorning Thursday, the day after the biopsy, I had immersed myself in work at school and temporarily lost track of time. I had forgotten the hospital's pledge to give us the pathology results that afternoon.

Student editors, between classes, had congregated in the newsroom, checking their e-mail, assigning news coverage, and mapping out the next day's newspaper. My office was inside the newsroom, and I had an open-door policy. That meant I had little privacy and even less peace and quiet when students were there.

Even though the newspaper's forty-five staff members weren't all in the newsroom at the same time, the spacious, open area frequently became hectic.

A telephone on the sports desk rang repeatedly.

"Someone answer that phone!" an editor barked.

An emergency dispatcher's voice crackled over the police scanner: "Possible signal eighty-seven at McDonald's on Lindsey . . . Do you copy, twenty-two?"

"Ten-four, dispatch. I'm on my way," an officer responded.

A reporter was puzzled.

"What's an eighty-seven?" she asked an editor.

"A drunk."

CNN and Fox talking heads spouted their latest news updates, adding to the commotion.

"Martha Stewart has just signed up for her own version of *The Apprentice* on NBC," a Fox commentator announced. "She'll get at least $100,000 an episode, the same as . . ."

Then my phone rang. It was Becky, a pleasant interruption for me from grading class assignments and red-marking the newspaper for mistakes.

Her voice was particularly warm and kind, not her usual sexy self. She sounded innocent and vulnerable and soothing.

"How's your day going?" she asked.

"Fine."

We shared our morning for a minute or two, and the conversation trailed off.

"The radiologist called with the biopsy results," she said.

"I thought they weren't supposed to call until this afternoon."

"They got the results early, and she called me," Becky said, and then she paused. I was still struggling with my absent-mindedness when she spoke again.

"It's cancer."

I didn't say anything. I sat silently holding the phone to my ear. I couldn't think of anything to say. The moment seemed forever. Her words had confirmed what I already knew. The newsroom sounds distanced themselves, and my mind drifted off to another place, another time, twenty years earlier.

I thought of the first time I saw Becky, standing in front of the savings and loan building waiting for our blind date. She looked as if she couldn't be more than seventeen years old. Her waist-length red hair glistened in the noonday sun. Her green eyes sparkled like life itself. She was as radiant a creature as I had ever seen.

As if it were yesterday, I thought of that first date, the first time I held her hand, the first time I kissed her, the first time I caressed her, and the boundless love that flourished from it all. Her strength, her spirit, her very being, was a gift to me from God.

I was blessed, I thought, regardless of what was to come.

"Are you okay?"

The sound of Becky's voice refocused my thoughts.

"I'm fine," I said. "I thought it was probably cancer."

Our words were subdued.

"We'll beat this thing," she said.

"I know."

"We have to."

We said our good-byes and hung up.

Almost as soon as I put the phone down, it rang again. Dr. Connally was calling to apologize and to reschedule my Monday appointment.

"I'm sorry you had to hear the biopsy results from someone else," he said. "I didn't know the hospital was going to call you. I prefer to tell my patients myself."

"That's fine," I said. "They called Becky, and she called me."

Dr. Connally wanted to see Becky and me at 4:30 that afternoon rather than waiting until Monday. He said he would explain everything that was going to happen to me.

"I'll see you two this afternoon," he said, and hung up.

My mind turned to mush. I couldn't think straight. I hadn't planned what I needed to do if the pathology report came back positive. I guess I was in denial. Even though I had suspected the tumor was malignant, I had done nothing to prepare.

I shuffled and reorganized the papers I was grading into a neat stack. I moved the red-marked newspaper aside. I sat quietly for a few minutes, trying to collect myself. My mind swirled with jumbled thoughts of what I needed to do next. I had to tell my boss first. I walked down the hall toward the business office, still unsure of what I was going to say to her.

Twila Smith, the director of Student Media, was alone. I tapped on the door with my knuckles and invited myself in, as I always did. She looked up and smiled.

"What's up, Jack?"

I looked at her for a moment, not knowing what to say first.

"I'm going to have to take next week off," I said.

She looked at me quizzically.

"I've got breast cancer."

She winced. "Oh, no!" Her smile turned to anguish.

"I have to have surgery next Tuesday."

"I'm so sorry," she said.

Her initial shock subsided, and we talked as if we were family. I had worked closely with her since I came to OU in 1993. I related how I had discovered my little nodule seven months earlier; how I had put it in the back of my mind, choosing to ignore it; how the biopsy had come about. I explained what I expected to happen the following week.

She asked how I was doing and how Becky was taking it.

"Is there anything I can do? Do you need anything?"

"I don't know. Look after the newsroom, I guess."

"Do you want me to teach your class while you're gone?"

"That would help a lot. I wouldn't have to get someone from the college."

"Would you like me to tell the newsroom staff?"

"No, I'll do it."

Twila was compassionate and caring. That was her nature. I appreciated her, and she made me feel comfortable talking about the cancer.

I went back to my office, sat down behind my desk, and looked at the assignments still needing to be graded. I picked up my favorite ballpoint and resumed critiquing. I scribbled across the first paper I read: "Weak lead." I pointed out editorializing in the second graph and noted the difference between "its" and "it's" in the third. But my mind wasn't on grading.

I didn't tell anyone else, either in Student Media or in the journalism college, about my cancer. That was strange for me. I usually told everyone I saw everything I knew. This situation seemed different somehow—private, something I wasn't ready to share. I didn't know why. I just didn't want to talk about it.

No doubt, I had already begun to put up my emotional defenses, retreating into my shell and reverting to that reclusive place I had gone all my life when fear of the unknown threatened me.

I went home about 4 o'clock to pick up Becky. On the way to the appointment with Dr. Connally,

Becky said she knew I had cancer when we left the hospital after the biopsy the day before.

"I'm not sure if it was a gut feeling or watching the nurses act so consoling with you," she said.

"Yeah, they were nice."

"When I had my mammogram, they weren't very personable."

"Really?"

"When they gave us all those pamphlets on breast cancer, I knew."

"I didn't think about that."

Becky had asked the radiologist to call her at home with the pathology results so she could call me at work. When our phone rang at home, she looked at the caller ID.

"I just froze," she said.

The doctor told her about the cancer. She had no questions.

"I just hung up the phone and cried like a big baby."

Becky called Patti, Dr. Bill's wife. Patti told her to go ahead and cry, get it out of her system, and then call me.

I never saw Becky cry during the entire ordeal. She hid her emotions. She would hide the fact that she cried in the shower over the next few days. But I knew how she felt. She felt exactly as I would have felt if she were the one who had just been diagnosed with cancer.

"I wanted to stay strong for you," she told me later. "I didn't want you to see me cry."

Her thinking she had to hide her emotions made me sad. I was so used to her strength, her fearlessness, and her deal-with-it attitude that sometimes I didn't recognize how much she was hurting, how much she concealed her feelings.

Becky was the rock in our family. I remembered our cocker spaniel puppy falling into the swimming pool in Muskogee. I looked out the kitchen window and saw something bobbing under the winter pool cover. Becky shot out the back door and rescued the pup while I was still standing in the kitchen trying to get my wits about me. She was one of those people who instinctively reacted in a crisis.

Becky, like me, worried that the cancer had spread to other parts of my body. She assured me she would be okay if anything happened to me. I was twelve years older, and I had always assumed I would die first. We had talked about death. She said the best scenario would be to die together because we loved each other so much, but she knew that would kill Stephanie.

She called me a survivor.

"God has a plan for you," she said. "Maybe this is just a hurdle."

Becky's mom, Mary, had lost her struggle with lung cancer four months and two chemotherapy treatments after her diagnosis. The disease and chemotherapy left an indelible impression on Becky.

"Chemotherapy kills people," she said after Mary died. "I'll never have chemo."

She had tempered that notion over the years: "Every time you turn around, you're talking to a breast cancer survivor." Treatment had come a long way in seven years.

Still, I knew my diagnosis had to petrify her. She resigned herself to taking one day at a time. Both of us did. She said she wasn't going to dwell on anything but positive thoughts. I knew she would trade places with me in a heartbeat. She knew I was scared.

Becky was a firm believer that God didn't give you any more than you could handle. "Apparently we can handle a hell of a lot," she said.

She said she put her faith in the Lord and knew that He would take care of us.

I did too. My faith was strong.

Becky especially dreaded telling Stephanie about the diagnosis. She phoned Chap, Steph's husband, ahead of time to let him know she would call Stephanie at home when he was with her. That backfired. Stephanie called Becky first.

"I couldn't lie to her," Becky said.

Stephanie's only experience with cancer was when her grandmother struggled with lung cancer.

"Everyone always said chemo killed Me-maw," Stephanie said. "I never thought that."

She thought the cancer and Mary's health caused her to die.

"That's not going to happen to you," Stephanie said. "Grandparents die, but your parents don't."

Children think that their parents are inde-structible, that they're never going to die.

I had always been there for Steph the past twenty years, and she thought I always would be. Nevertheless, she was beginning to realize that Becky and I wouldn't always be with her.

Stephanie had worked in a psychiatric unit at an Oklahoma City hospital for a while. Her office was on the same floor as the oncology unit. She could see the room full of people taking chemo treatments. She told me about a man who spent every day at the hospital, visiting the other patients.

"In the psych unit, we had cancer survivors," she said. "Maybe God was preparing me."

Becky and I arrived at Dr. Connally's office at 4:30 sharp. A nurse ushered us into an examination room and said the doctor would be with us in a minute. I sat on the bed at the foot of the examination table, and Becky took the only chair in the room.

The wait wasn't long, unusual for a doctor's office. The door opened, and Dr. Connally briskly entered the room. He smiled as he greeted us, and we shook hands. He pulled up a stool and sat in front of us.

I liked Dr. Connally. So did Becky. He was direct, no-bones-about-it, honest.

On Tuesday, when he first examined me and ordered the biopsy, he'd said I had no choice but to have surgery, regardless of whether the tumor was malignant. The tumor had to come out. I too knew

I had no choice. I knew I had to go through whatever was necessary to get rid of the disease. My treatment would mean surgery, chemotherapy, and radiation.

Once the biopsy revealed the tumor was malignant, I wanted the thing out of my body, and the quicker the better. I felt that as long as it was in my breast, it was festering and probably spreading the disease to other parts of my body. The tumor had already moved away from the nipple where I discovered it back in June.

I quickly put my trust in Dr. Connally. I generally trusted professionals until they gave me a reason not to. That was probably not a typical journalistic mind-set, but it was mine. Dr. Connally knew about cancer. I didn't. I had no inclination to take a crash course in medicine or alternative approaches before I decided what to do. What he said made sense to me. I didn't view the mastectomy any differently from a surgery to remove a tumor in my stomach or in my brain, if that's where the cancer had been. No doubt, my reasoning differed from how a woman might approach breast surgery.

I had talked with my friend Dr. Bill and my family physician, Dr. Lindsey. I also knew the hospital had a cancer consultation committee of doctors and specialists who collaborated on a patient's treatment plan. I was ready to do what Dr. Connally recommended.

At our meeting Thursday, the surgeon thoroughly explained the treatment plan we would follow. He referred me to the National Comprehensive Cancer Network website, which was cosponsored by the American Cancer Society and provided surgeon and patient guidelines for treatment. It was informative and easy to understand, a must-read for cancer patients and their families.

I'd already visited the National Comprehensive Cancer Network website, which showed five stages—0, I, II, III, and IV. Stage IV, known as metastatic, was the most advanced. It meant cancer had spread from the breast and lymph nodes under the arm to other areas of the body such as the liver, lungs, bones, and brain. The stage was important to doctors in determining the best treatment. It was important to me too, for helping to gauge the seriousness of my plight.

Dr. Connally told us about sentinel node mapping, a procedure in which the surgeon finds and removes the sentinel node—the first lymph node into which a tumor drains and the one most likely to contain cancer cells. If he could find that sentinel node during surgery, it would give him a better idea of whether any cancer had spread.

If the sentinel node was "hot," he said he might have to remove all of the lymph nodes under my right arm. That could cause a condition known as lymphedema. When the lymph nodes are removed, it causes an inability to excrete sweat under the arms, and a buildup of fluids can cause the arm to swell—and to remain that way. I would have to be extremely careful not to scratch, cut, or damage my right arm in any way for the rest of my life. I couldn't risk infection in that arm. Vaccinations, IVs, blood pressure checks—all would have to be administered on my left arm.

During the course of my treatment, I came to dread lymphedema more than the cancer itself. This possibility terrified me. It threatened the very things I loved to do most, and I couldn't get it out of my mind. How could I give up physical activity, landscaping, planting, the satisfying and relaxing things that Becky and I loved to do together? It would affect my right arm too. I was right-handed, and I typed for a living. My pulse raced.

I tried to concentrate on what the doctor was telling us, but he related a lot of information in a very few minutes. My brain's processing ability reached overload. I couldn't think clearly.

Even Becky didn't ask questions, and that was rare. She was uncommonly curious—like a good reporter—and usually cross-examined doctors relentlessly. But she did take notes while Dr. Connally explained the process. A time or two, he looked over her shoulder to make sure she got everything correct. Neither Becky nor I knew what questions to ask. We were ignorant about cancer and its treatment, and we were still reeling from the diagnosis.

Just before Dr. Connally left the room, he gave us one more opportunity for questions. I had one.

"You are a good doctor, aren't you?" I asked with a straight face.

He grinned and said he was the best.

Becky and I drove home apprehensive, dazed, overwhelmed, angry, and scared.

4
BREAST CANCER
A Woman's Disease

When most people think of breast cancer, they think of Eve, not Adam. Like most men and women, I didn't realize men could contract what is widely considered a woman's disease. When most people think of a mastectomy, they think of a woman's breast, not a man's.

I knew very little about breast cancer, except that it occurred in women and it had deadly consequences. In fact, I knew very little about cancer. My late sister in Tennessee had survived uterine cancer in the eighties, and my sister Inabelle's husband, Charles, had died of brain cancer in the sixties. I idolized Charles. He and my sister, against my parents' better judgment, of course, had given me my first real gun, a Red Ryder BB rifle.

I remembered Charles, my sister, and I eating lunch at a Red Lion roast beef restaurant in St.

Louis, where they lived. Doctors had given Charles six months to live. As he ate, food dripped from his mouth down his chin. He never realized it. My sister tenderly wiped the food from his face. I was young, and that image of cancer stuck with me.

Inabelle practically raised me during my formative years because my mother and dad worked at the family produce business six, sometimes seven, days a week. When she married and moved away, I was only five. I was so upset that my mother agreed to let me spend a week or two each summer with Inabelle and Charles.

For entertainment when they lived in Dallas, we parked near the tarmac at Love Field and watched the planes take off and land. When they lived at Guymon, in the desolate Oklahoma Panhandle, there was nothing to do. At night, Charles chauffeured us out of town and across the arid plains. I delighted in watching as the headlights illuminated jackrabbits and tumbleweeds streaking across the prairie in front of us. When I visited them in Broken Arrow, a suburb of Tulsa, I used to lie awake late at night and listen to the lonesome wail of a train. We didn't have trains in Tahlequah, where I grew up, and the sound fascinated me.

Inabelle entertained me during the day. She baked oatmeal cookies with walnuts. She scribbled line drawings of horses on typing paper. I couldn't draw horses, but she was good at it. Sometimes, she drew three or four galloping stallions to a page. I penciled in the saddles and bridles and sagebrush and then drew Gene Autry and his deputies atop the horses. I colored the drawings with crayons that Inabelle always had on hand for my visits.

I saw my mother in Inabelle. In a lot of ways, she was my mother.

I never thought I would get cancer. As a baby, I had pneumonia and wasn't expected to live. As a teenager, I tested positive for tuberculosis. My mother's stories about the infant illness and the TB test, which turned out to be a false positive due to scar tissue from the pneumonia, caused me to believe I had weak lungs. I had always thought that when I died, it would probably come courtesy of lung disease, such as emphysema.

Breast cancer was so rare among men that when the federal government passed a law related to the disease in 1998, it was known as the Women's Health and Cancer Rights Act. Legislators intended to make insurance companies provide certain mastectomy-related benefits. No doubt, the act required insurance companies to cover men under this act too, but my story made the name seem ironic.

I could have told our lawmakers that men got breast cancer too. Former U.S. senator Edward W. Brooke of Massachusetts probably already had told them. When Brooke found out he had breast cancer, he began speaking publicly to bring attention to a disease many men assumed they could not get.

Consider this Mother Goose rhyme, copyrighted in 1916:

> What are little boys made of, made of?
> What are little boys made of?
> "Snaps and snails, and puppy-dogs' tails;
> And that's what little boys are made of."

> What are little girls made of, made of?
> What are little girls made of?
> "Sugar and spice, and all that's nice;
> And that's what little girls are made of."

The sugar-and-spice theory—the gender-based concept that girls were treated and behaved one way and that boys were treated and behaved another way—was alive and well. To address some of these misconceptions, First Lady Laura Bush was pushing an initiative aimed at adolescent boys. In a May 2005 *Ladies Home Journal* article, Bush said she wanted to get people thinking about how we treated boys, how we assigned stereotypes. Boys didn't cry and they didn't show emotion. Bush said we weren't teaching boys the life skills we taught girls. We hadn't given boys words to be emotional, to have an emotional life.

Society's mores and stereotypes, perpetuated since the beginning of humankind, had influenced emotions and the way men and women physically looked at their bodies—and at each other's bodies. They affected the way we thought, the way we talked, the way we interacted.

Men thought differently about their breasts and women's breasts. A man thought nothing of talking about his testicles. He was a man. He had balls. The essence of man was testosterone. His self-image, his machismo, his psyche, his very manhood were at stake. Men didn't cry, and they didn't like men who did.

You wouldn't hear a man talk about his breasts. He may have spoken disparagingly about the man-boobies on another man, but the only time he would mention breasts was when they were on a woman. Some women had difficulty talking about breast cancer, but most men didn't talk about it at all.

Stephanie called me a week after my surgery. She was upset. She related a telephone conversation she'd had after telling a friend about my cancer.

"Well, breast cancer has got to be worse for women," the woman told Stephanie. "Women are more into their breasts, and breasts are more about who women are than men."

I was offended by that opinion, too, at first. After I thought about it, though, I realized the woman was probably right. I didn't worry about having breast cancer. I worried about having cancer.

Stephanie thought the fact that the illness was stereotyped as a woman's disease certainly didn't make it any easier for a man.

"They all go through the same things: finding the lump, having the biopsy, surgery, chemotherapy, and radiation," she said.

At work, I had a split appointment, which meant I had two supervisors. Half my salary came from the journalism college, and the dean, a man, was my supervisor. The other half of my paycheck came from Student Media, a nonacademic department in Student Affairs, and a woman was my supervisor.

I received totally different reactions to my diagnosis from my male boss and my female boss. The dean, who was great to work for and professional, never came to see me in my office or called me on the phone or e-mailed me to see how I was doing after the diagnosis. The woman supervisor came to my office every day and asked how I was doing. She called my wife to check on my condition when I was off work for three days for the mastectomy. She came to the hospital, along with my former Student Media boss, Susan Sasso, while I was in surgery.

I reacted to them differently too, based on their gender. I went to the woman's office immediately after Becky called to tell me the tumor was malignant. I never went to my male boss to tell him about my diagnosis. Ever.

Friday, the day after I learned my diagnosis, I attended a meeting in the new journalism building. After that, Fred Blevens, the associate dean, and I walked across the oval to my building for a publications board meeting. The moment seemed right to me, and I just blurted out, "Fred, I've got breast cancer."

Before he could respond, I explained that I already had a contingency plan for my classes. I was alone with Fred on the oval, and he was a good friend. I didn't realize I might shock him. I was inconsiderate and insensitive to his emotions.

"Jack, I don't know what to say," he said. I guess I didn't either.

I don't know how I expected the dean to know I was ill. I guess I assumed Fred would tell him, though I didn't ask him to.

My intention is not to insinuate that anyone should have done anything differently, but to make a point. Men reacted differently than women.

Men have difficulty talking to other men about their health problems, and even more so when the affliction is considered a woman's. When some men first learned about my breast cancer, a half-grin, half-smirk crossed their face, just for an instant.

I never picked up on that reaction in women. They seemed more empathetic, gentler, more like I would expect them to respond if I had told them I had heart disease or any other serious illness. Perhaps my own stereotypes caused me to anticipate a different reaction from men. Perhaps women identified with my plight more readily than men.

Just about every man who knew I had breast cancer asked how I found the tumor. The nuclear medicine tech asked. Doctors and nurses asked. Men at work asked. Even the barber asked. No doubt, they thought if it could happen to me, it could happen to them.

Their asking about the tumor made me feel important in an odd sort of way. It was like, as a kid, winning a blue ribbon with my steer at the livestock show, and all the other competitors wanting to know what I fed the calf. It made me believe I had information about breast cancer that other people would like to know, especially if they had been recently diagnosed or they wanted to learn how to support a loved one or a friend who had cancer.

5

THE WAITING GAME

Becky and I watched TV the night we learned about the surgery. We kept pretty much to ourselves. The evening didn't seem out of the ordinary, a little quieter perhaps.

I didn't feel emotional. I suppose I had already resigned myself to my predicament, or it was the calm before the storm. Becky and I had talked ourselves out the past two days, anyway. I felt like I had very little, if any, control over my life. I downshifted my nerves. I withdrew. I internalized. I put my life in God's hands. And I waited.

Becky and I had planned to go to my sister Inabelle's retirement home in Oklahoma City on Saturday. She was eighty-three. I wanted to tell her my news in person. I thought my diagnosis would have an adverse effect on her, since her husband had died of brain cancer. She had lived alone for nearly fifty years after Charles died, never caring to date or re-marry. She seemed to have never let him go.

Becky and I went to bed. I slept until 3 A.M., and then lay awake trying to take it all in. At that point, I decided I didn't want to tell my students about the cancer after all. I wanted my boss to do it. I didn't want to see the look in their eyes if they didn't care, and if they did care, I thought it would be too emotional for me to handle.

I felt confident the surgery would go okay, but I feared the surgeons would find cancer in my lymph nodes and that it had already spread throughout my body. I don't remember ever talk-ing to anyone about that. I didn't want to talk about it. I didn't want to talk about what scared me the most. Perhaps I should have. Instead, I franti-cally prayed to God that the cancer hadn't already infiltrated my bloodstream and infected other or-gans, and that it wouldn't.

I didn't want to go through what Charles did. I didn't want a doctor telling me that I had six months to live and then facing an indignant and unmerciful death. Sometimes you don't know what to think, what to do. I had never faced any-thing like this. I didn't know the best course of ac-tion. I didn't have a reference point. Cancer had snuck up on me. Since I didn't realize the disease was in my breast, common sense told me that it was possibly eating away at me in other places.

I looked over at Becky asleep beside me, and I felt the wonder of her. I thanked God for my bless-ings, for a wonderful life, and for bringing her and

Stephanie into my world. They had loved, comforted, and fulfilled me. They had brought me a lifetime of joy in twenty years. If He intended for me to die, I would have few regrets.

My mind churned with logic and fact. I wasn't particularly worried about who would provide financially for Becky. We had already taken care of that. We had saved enough for her to live out her life, and she was still young. She could work if she wanted. We had paid off the house mortgage, we had life insurance, and we didn't have any debt.

She had a family support system nearby, something I felt was important. Becky and Steph were still uncommonly close fifteen years after Steph left the nest. She and her husband Chap lived forty minutes away in Edmond, on the north side of Oklahoma City. Becky's two sisters, Francie and Gigi, lived two and a half hours away.

My unquestioned faith assured me that God would watch over Becky and take care of her for me. I knew God and I trusted His infinite wisdom and His promise of eternal life. I believed my life was in order.

What I feared most that night, what I couldn't bear to think about, was what I would miss if I were not there with Becky. I wanted to see her even happier and more content after a life's journey that had been too hard on her. I couldn't imagine her shopping for clothes, something she loved to do, without me there; or her planting daffodils and tulips and manicuring the yard without my help. I couldn't imagine her browsing the outlet malls and shops in Branson without me walking hand in hand with her.

I couldn't imagine her in bed without me lying beside her. I couldn't stand the thought of never seeing her again, never hearing her voice again, never holding her again, never kissing her again, never making love with her again.

I wanted to see Stephanie and Chap grow in so many ways together. I wanted to see their successes in life and to help them when they struggled. I wanted to hear about their sailing exploits, their skiing adventures, and their dinner parties, and to see them move into a larger house with a grand swimming pool and a garage with enough room for Chap to use his tools and build incredible things. I wanted to see their children someday, because the two of them would make great parents.

I realized that it was selfish to think of what I wanted or what I would miss, but I knew Becky and Stephanie. They would grieve, and they would survive.

Even as a child in the 1940s, I always worried that I would miss out on something. My mom and dad reared a litter of seven, born in the twenties, thirties, and forties, when rural families were larger. I was the baby, seven years younger than my youngest sibling. I was underfoot every time my mother moved or I thought she was going somewhere without me.

I cried myself to sleep on nights when my parents went to the movie theater and wouldn't let me go. It wasn't that I cared about the movie, because

I was too young to understand most movies anyway. I just wanted to go somewhere—anywhere.

When Becky went somewhere, I still had the desire to tag along. I suppose that childhood urge, that insatiable curiosity about where my parents were going, that nomad quality, drove me to become a journalist. I wanted to know what was down the road, what was on the other side of the mountain. I wanted to know what was going on there. I wanted to know things before anybody else knew. And then I wanted to be the first to tell someone.

I was the first person in Muskogee to learn that Richard Nixon had resigned. I was working the wire machine when the Associated Press sent out the flash alert, AP's highest priority for news before computers and the Internet took over the world. "Nixon resigns," the flash read. I kept the piece of teletype paper with the words on it.

Nothing excited me more than covering a raging fire in a downtown Muskogee furniture store or a rampaging flood on the Arkansas River. I drove my GMC Jimmy a half mile through two feet of water gushing across Smith Ferry Road. I feared I would get washed off into the ditch before I reached the Meadows subdivision and the real flood. I prayed the engine wouldn't flood out. News still got my adrenaline pumping. How I would miss the excitement of living!

Lying awake in the stillness late at night became a time to think. It was so peaceful then, with the only interruption the occasional hoot of a solitary horned owl. Over and over I thought about what I needed to do. The only certainty was the uncertainty of it all.

Anxiety was again becoming a way of life for me. My anxiety this time was different, though, not like what I experienced with Sandra, my first wife. My apprehension and edginess over her became so intense at times that my skin would crawl. In an instant, I would feel as if goose bumps or hives covered my skin. We could be sitting in a restaurant, and if Sandra heard a baby cry, her emotions would explode. She couldn't stand the thought of somebody mistreating a baby. I knew that so well that eventually every time I heard a baby cry, my defenses reared up and my skin squirmed—just like the conditioned reflexes Pavlov had found. I was so fearful of what Sandra might do next.

My skin didn't crawl as a result of my anxiety about the cancer, but I lived with fear of the unknown from the beginning of my ordeal to the end. I tried not to think about the disease, the surgery, the chemotherapy, or the radiation. I tried to go on with my routine as if everything were normal, but everything resembling normal was gone.

Those fears lingered close to my consciousness, and they haunted me from the time I was diagnosed until my treatment ended. At times I couldn't think of anything else. I tried not to let the apprehension overwhelm me, but sometimes in the stillness late at night, my emotions took control and pushed me into the abyss of my own fears.

I would wake up, restless, and my mind would begin to churn. I couldn't stop thinking about what might happen to me. Had the cancer spread? Would all of my lymph nodes have to be removed? How many do I have anyway? Would I get lymphedema? Would chemotherapy make me sick? How sick? Could I still work? Would I survive?

Becky and I drove to Inabelle's retirement home apartment in Oklahoma City on Friday afternoon instead of waiting for the weekend. Becky had called Inabelle to tell her we were coming and that we had some news.

Inabelle was excited to see us. She mistakenly thought our news was that my late sister Doris's probate case in Tennessee had been settled. She thought we were bringing her a check from the estate, and her disappointment showed. My news didn't affect her the way I thought it might. She listened to me and acknowledged what I was saying, but she never engaged. It occurred to me that I could have called her on the phone and saved the eighty-mile round-trip.

Her reaction reminded me of the day I told my eighty-eight-year-old dad I was going to marry Becky. He promptly changed the subject and never mentioned it again. I guess he assumed I was on the rebound and this marriage wouldn't last. It was too soon. He forgot I was forty-four years old at the time, and I knew exactly what I wanted.

When we left, Inabelle didn't mention the cancer. She called the next day to apologize for not wishing me luck with my surgery.

Stephanie and Chap came to Norman on Friday night. As soon as Steph walked in the front door, she half smiled at me, and then her expression saddened. She hugged my neck and began to cry. It was difficult to keep my composure. I usually cried when she cried. I told her crying was okay. She cried on the way to our house and on the way home.

"I felt so helpless," she told me later. "All I could do was cry." She told me how she fell apart at work. She had to cancel her counseling sessions with clients because she didn't think she could help them. Counselors learned early in their education that if they couldn't take care of themselves, they couldn't help anyone else.

The Sunday before surgery was a day in slow motion. I turned on the CD player and punched in a favorite, Josh Groban. I could barely hear the sound as the music began, and then softly, slowly the crescendo of Groban's voice, magnified by surround sound, resonated through the living room.

Emotion swept over me, and I had the same feeling of despair as I did when Sandra died suddenly in the spring of 1985. For weeks after I lost her, I listened to the classical music we had enjoyed together. I couldn't shake my grief. I couldn't concentrate. I couldn't sleep. I couldn't stop thinking about her. The music accentuated my feelings of love and loneliness and loss. Finally, I had to give up Tchaikovsky and Prokofiev and Debussy or lose myself.

My heart grieved just as it had twenty years earlier. Tears streaked down my face. Once again, music enraptured me, and Groban's lyrics brought memories of Sandra flooding back.

> When you say you love me
> The world goes still, so still inside and
> When you say you love me
> For a moment, there's no one else alive.

Music—any kind of beautiful music—could touch me when I felt good, and it could crush me when I didn't. Music therapy could change a person's mood for the better—but not mine, not on that day. I had to say good-bye to Josh Groban for a while. I turned off the CD player.

Becky and I went to bed early that evening, both wondering what was to come.

I wished I had insisted the first surgeon biopsy that pea-size nodule in June during my first visit. I wished I had taken the initiative to schedule a follow-up visit whether the lump grew or not. I wished I had known more about cancer.

I wished I hadn't been so clueless. If you find a nodule and your doctor says not to worry about it, get a second opinion. Don't wait, as I did, for the thing to grow. If the doctor tells you cancer is hard and fixed, don't believe him. That's a myth. If you find something and your doctor drags his feet about a biopsy or about testing, find a new doctor.

I wished I had known what I was doing while I was in the shower. I wished I had been consciously looking for something, intentionally examining myself, but I wasn't. I was just plain lucky. By mere chance, I felt something out of the ordinary and had sense enough to go to the doctor. After the fact, I realized how critical early detection and self-examination are to surviving cancer.

Most women check themselves. I never thought about examining myself for breast cancer. I'm a guy, right? My suggestion for men is to take a page from the women's good-sense manual. Examine yourself. Schedule medical checkups at least annually. I didn't do that. If you think you can't get cancer, you're wrong. If you think a man can't get breast cancer, you're wrong. Cancer develops over time. I read somewhere that if you live long enough, you're going to get cancer. The disease arises from a complex mixture of lifestyle, heredity, and environment. If you think it won't happen to you, ask yourself: "Can I afford to take that risk?"

Educate yourself, not just so you can take care of yourself, but so you can support family and friends who may need your help should they become victims.

Less than one percent of the male population contracts breast cancer. I didn't know that. The average age of a man diagnosed with breast cancer is sixty-three. I didn't know that, either, but when I discovered my tumor, I was sixty-three.

Reduce stress. I let the Tennessee probate ordeal increase my stress level. I should have chilled out. I believed that stress played a significant role in causing cancer, but there was no scientific evidence of that. Researchers, though, had not ruled out a possible connection between stress, the immune system, and cancer. If stress didn't cause cancer, I believed it inhibited the immune system from fighting the cancer. Obviously, I was not educated in medicine, but common sense told me stress played a role in cancer, just as it did in other illnesses.

Consult the National Comprehensive Cancer Network at www.nccn.org. Its treatment guidelines for patients helped inform me and allay my fears.

Confide in someone if you think you're in trouble. Men aren't as aware of their bodies as women are, and consequently men don't take care of themselves as they should. Guys may not like the doctor's poking and prodding, but it sure beats the alternative.

6
THE MASTECTOMY

On the night before surgery, Becky had to take three ibuprofen pills to help her sleep. I slept fine. I didn't know whether I was exhausted from fretting the previous five days, or whether I just wanted the surgery over with. Probably both.

We got up early, due at the hospital at 6 A.M. We waited for Steph to get to the house so we could all go together. Becky said she felt like she was in a fog. I felt nervous.

Becky worried about me and wanted to protect me. I had never been in the hospital except for kidney stones. I had never had an operation. She thought I was naive, and I suppose I was.

The waiting room was crowded for so early in the morning. There were so many patients, fifteen to twenty, preparing for surgery. I was surprised. I hadn't expected so many. I thought we'd gotten up early, but the room was nearly full when we arrived.

I had difficulty distinguishing patients from their relatives and friends. Most of the people looked like they had just rolled out of bed, thrown on some clothes, and headed for the hospital. No doubt they did. That was what I did. Most of them were seniors. Only one man appeared to be in his twenties.

Becky fidgeted. It was cold in the waiting room. She pulled her coat tighter around her shoulders. The room seemed bare and sterile. Artificial trees and greenery failed to soften the surroundings. The chairs, with leather pads and chrome arms and legs, were hard and uncomfortable.

A nurse called my name, and the two of us left Becky and Stephanie behind. The nurse escorted me into the operating prep area. She asked if I needed to go to the bathroom. I did. I had already gone at home, and then when we entered the hospital lobby. I needed to go again. Obviously, I was nervous. The nurse tossed me a gown and told me to take off my clothes.

I remembered to take off my socks and underwear, something I'd failed to do during my first stay in a hospital, Muskogee Regional, thirteen years earlier when I had a lithotripsy procedure to remove a kidney stone.

The nurse checked my blood pressure and pulse and showed me a machine that looked like a Shop-Vac with a plastic blanket attached to its hose. She pulled the air blanket over me and said someone later would inflate it with warm air. Studies showed that patients kept warm prior to surgery fared much better during the operation and were less prone to infection after surgery. The nurse said the surgery wasn't scheduled for a couple of hours.

I asked her about lymphedema, the condition Dr. Connally had told me sometimes occurs when surgeons remove the lymph nodes. I was obsessed with that side effect. She explained the symptoms again and said it was "god-awful ugly." Sorry I asked.

I needed to go to the bathroom again.

A nurse brought Becky and Stephanie to the pre-op room. I was glad. I had missed them already. I didn't like waiting by myself. Stephanie wanted to know what the Shop-Vac was.

Becky said her sisters, Gigi and Francie, were on their way from Muskogee to Norman. She said they didn't want me to go into surgery until they got to the hospital. Becky later said she was thinking: "How in the hell am I going to stop the surgery until they get here?"

Becky was the youngest sister. Growing up, she was the tomboy, the freckle-faced redhead with bad eyes, thick glasses, and long, skinny legs. Gi, the oldest, was the beautiful brunette. Francie, the cheerleader, had the tan, the blond hair, the body, and the boyfriends.

Becky excelled in sports. She roller-skated in public shows, and she won the city's junior bowling championship. As the pitcher on her summer-league softball team, she never lost a game in three years. She ran track. She quarterbacked the junior girls against the senior girls in the high school's powder-puff football game.

Even as an adult, second was never good enough for her. She had to be number one in whatever she did. She played in the city's softball league and coached little girls' softball. She was competitive, assertive, intelligent. She was the leader, the sister everyone looked to. Her dad even solicited her advice.

Shortly after I married her, we took Stephanie for an afternoon of softball practice. I'd never seen Becky play. She was batting, Stephanie was pitching, and I was shagging fly balls. I stood forty feet behind Stephanie, waiting for my petite wife to hit the first pitch. Becky motioned for me to move back. I moved back thirty feet. She motioned again.

"Move back!"

"Yeah, right," I thought. But to appease her, I moved back another thirty feet to deep center field.

Becky swatted the first pitch. The ball cleared Stephanie's head by a mile and kept rising and rising—into the sun. I backpedaled. The fly ball sailed ten feet over my head and dropped just short of the center field fence.

"My God, what a slugger," I thought.

I never again doubted Becky's sports prowess. Not even when she told me her bowling average was 185.

The longer we waited in the pre-op room, the more apprehensive and antsy Becky became. She wanted Gi and Francie to hurry. Fortunately for them, surgery was running behind schedule.

An aide pushed my bed, and me in it, to a room where a nurse stood ready to inject me with a radioactive substance that would help the doctor find the sentinel node. The aide said he wasn't supposed to let anyone come with me, but Becky could anyway. I figured he liked her red hair.

Karen Saunkeah—the nurse from the Breast Care Center, where I had the biopsy—prepared to inject me. I enjoyed seeing her familiar face, even if it was upside down. The only two times I saw her, I was lying down and she was standing over me. I recognized her anyway.

I still had lymphedema on my mind. Since Karen was a breast cancer survivor, I asked her if she minded answering personal questions. She didn't. Doctors had removed seven of her lymph nodes. They removed a four-centimeter tumor from her breast. My tumor was two centimeters, just less than an inch. Karen said her surgeon, like my first one, chose not to have a biopsy performed at the time she found her tumor. He didn't think it was cancer. Three years later, he biopsied the tumor and it was malignant.

I asked Karen how she handled lymphedema. She said she led a normal life. She wore gloves when working in the yard. If there was swelling, it wasn't permanent. Exercise and therapy combated it. She cautioned not to let anyone take my blood pressure or give an injection in my right arm. Her tumor was twice the size of mine; it had been growing in her breast three times as long as mine had grown in me, and she appeared in very good health.

Talking with someone who had gone through what I was about to go through helped me immensely. It changed my outlook, much more so than I would have thought. Her calming assurance quelled my anxiety and gave me confidence that everything would be all right even if I did contract lymphedema. I could still have a life after cancer.

I was one of those insecure people who needed a what-if plan—just in case. What would I do if this happened or that happened? As a Boy Scout, I had my what-if plans. What if the Russians invaded and occupied Cherokee County? What would I do? If I wanted to hide, where would I go? The answer was clear. Goats Bluff. It's a secluded, scenic place up the Illinois River from Tahlequah, the town where I grew up in eastern Oklahoma. My Boy Scout comrades and I had camped there many times. I felt safe from the Reds, knowing that Goats Bluff was there and that I had my plan. Nurse Karen gave me my what-if plan for lymphedema. I felt better about my situation already.

Patti and Stephanie were waiting when Becky and I returned from pre-op. We talked and waited for the call to surgery. The operating room chugged along an hour behind schedule as Becky's sisters arrived. As the six of us waited, I thought it didn't get much better: Five beautiful women surrounded me, and I was lying there in my gown without my socks and underwear.

An aide said it was time to go. He inflated the plastic blanket, and warmth surrounded me. He put another blanket over me and began rolling me down the hall toward the operating room, my entourage of women in tow. Stephanie kissed me on the cheek, and the other women hugged me and wished me good luck.

I began to think, a little belatedly perhaps, what if something happened during surgery? Things happen. My dad lived with a hernia for ten years, maybe longer, because he was afraid to go on the operating table. He feared he would never leave the hospital alive. He endured the pain rather than have the tear repaired. Eventually he either overcame his fear or the pain became too bad to bear. He allowed the operation, and he left the hospital alive.

I wasn't my dad. But I did have my own concerns. When someone was going to slice me open with a knife and poke around inside my chest, I didn't think it could be all that good. I had read how things went wrong in hospitals. Patients were admitted with minor problems, yet they died. Surgeons were given the wrong instructions and amputated the wrong leg.

Unsanitary conditions and a staph infection could kill a patient. I once had a staph infection that manifested itself as a boil inside my nose. It hurt so much I thought my face was going to fall off. I didn't want another staph infection, nor did I want my surgeon lopping off the wrong breast. I chose not to think about a cavalier saying we journalists had about making mistakes: "When journalists make a mistake, everybody knows about it, but when doctors make a mistake, they bury it."

In my mind, I knew the cancer could kill me, but in my heart, I knew it wouldn't. Perhaps I still thought I was invincible. Perhaps God still had things for me to do. Perhaps my survival instincts had kicked in.

Becky leaned over and kissed me on the lips. I watched her as the aide pushed me away. I tried to imprint her image—the way she looked at that very moment—in my brain.

A television tuned to a *CSI: Miami* rerun flickered as I waited for the anesthesiologist. An elderly woman in the bed next to me coughed up phlegm.

Her daughter, a short, stocky woman in her sixties, stepped closer to the bed with a box of Kleenex. Her voice was soothing, and she cooed over her mother's every whim. She wiped the old woman's mouth. She hovered, attentive, caring, as if she had sole responsibility for her mother's well-being. She anticipated her mother's every need, something an unknowing daughter wouldn't have been able to do.

The old woman coughed again and tried to clear her throat.

A nurse pulled the curtain separating the woman from me and whispered, "I'm sorry." I understood. I had phlegm occasionally myself.

I heard the mother's physician enter the room. The daughter raised her voice.

"Mama! The doctor's here!"

The daughter told the doctor he would have to speak loudly.

"You'll have to speak up!" the old woman repeated. "I can't hear very well."

"Hello!" the doctor said in a booming voice. "How are you feeling?"

"Huh? What'd he say?" the old woman asked.

"He asked how you're feeling," the daughter repeated.

As the old woman began telling the doctor her problems, my anesthesiologist came into the room. He explained the process that was about to happen to me. He said he would put the anesthetic into my IV, and I would go into the operating room soon. Surgery was backed up.

A nurse pushed the elderly woman's bed from behind the curtain toward the operating room. The double doors swung open.

"I'm 102 years old," the old woman piped up as her bed rolled through the doors. "Do you think I'll make it okay?"

The doors swung shut, and I never heard the answer.

Dr. Connally, in his scrubs, came out of the operating room and asked if I was ready. I was. He wanted to know if I had any questions. I didn't. He said it wouldn't be much longer. The anesthesiologist injected something into my IV.

I lost interest in *CSI: Miami* as a nurse began rolling my bed toward those double doors. I could only imagine what was in store for me. I thought of the old woman's last words: "Do you think I'll make it okay?"

My surgery brought back memories for Becky. In 1986, three months after we married, she started having stomach problems. Her doctor diagnosed the problem as an ulcer, the result of wedding jitters, a new job, moving to a different house, and meeting my family. The doctor performed an ultrasound to make sure she wasn't pregnant.

Becky wasn't pregnant. She had a baseball-size tumor attached to one of her ovaries. Fortunately, the tumor was benign. She had a hysterectomy. She said God answered the question we had talked about: Should we have children? This was His answer. Stephanie would be our only child.

In the early eighties, she bowled in a league. As she sat keeping score, she tilted her head to scratch it. She felt a knot on the right side of her skull. When she scratched, it hurt. Later that week while she was driving, horrible pains—like labor pains—suddenly shot through her head. She stopped and gripped the steering wheel. The pains lasted about thirty seconds.

Becky never seriously considered that her tumors might be malignant. Cancer wasn't that common in her world. She had no experience with it in her family. She didn't even tell her co-workers until the afternoon before the surgery. They reacted as you might expect, panic-stricken at first, but Becky still didn't worry much about it.

She was upset that nurses had cut off her waist-length hair and shaved one side of her head. She thought her hair was the only feminine part of her tomboyish looks.

A CAT scan discovered two tumors inside her skull. The neurosurgeon couldn't decide if they were growing toward the brain or out toward the skull. The uncertainty made surgery more dangerous. Once the neurosurgeon began the process, he found the tumors were growing out of her skull. He removed them, and lab tests revealed they were benign.

After the surgery, she had a splitting headache. Eventually, she found the cause. Surgeons had wrapped her head in bandages, with only holes for her eyes and mouth. Nurses had braided her remaining hair into twenty-five little braids. When they wrapped her head so tight, it pulled her hair.

Because of an infection, surgeons couldn't put a filler in her skull, so they used screws. She laughed when somebody told her she had a screw loose.

"You're in the recovery room," a voice said. "Are you awake?"

Later I couldn't remember those next few minutes. A nurse was asking me something. The next thing I knew, Becky was leaning over kissing me.

Postoperative patients lay in beds lining both sides of the room, much like cars angled in on either side of a dealership service area, some fixed for good and some probably not.

The hospital was full and I had to wait for a room on the third floor, so the nurses warehoused me downstairs for the afternoon. Dr. Bill and Patti came by and stayed for several hours. Chap arrived, and we camped in that small room until almost 6 o'clock.

Chap and Stephanie found the doctor's latex gloves. Chap grabbed one and blew it up. After tying the end in a knot, he drew a happy face on it and hung it from the light fixture. Kids, even young adults, had a way of lessening the stress level at the most opportune time.

I wasn't feeling any pain. I didn't think the morphine affected my mind. Becky said it did.

Finally, a nurse wheeled me up to the third floor—the cancer patient unit—and I settled in. Nurses checked my vital signs every hour. The first nurse checked me over, including my feet.

"Most nurses don't check your feet," Becky told me. "It's a good sign that she did."

"How come?"

"She was being thorough. If your feet are blue, it means you have a blood circulation problem."

Fortunately, my feet weren't blue.

Each nurse started to take my blood pressure in my right arm, since that was the side closest to the door. I remembered lymphedema and what Nurse Karen had said: Don't let anyone check your blood pressure or give you an injection in the right arm.

Becky suggested a nurse put a sign over the bed telling the other nurses not to use my right arm for the vitals check. The other nurses ignored the sign, of course, and kept trying to stick my right arm. Any kind of trauma or infection, any disruption of the skin, in my right arm could result in lymphedema.

Becky and Stephanie stood watch in the room all night. They went home early the next morning to freshen up.

The general surgeon who had initially examined me in June came by my room while they were gone. He had assisted Dr. Connally in the operating room. He said the pathology report was not complete, but the sentinel node and two other extracted lymph nodes tested negative.

The news overjoyed me. I tried to remember every word he said so I could report to Becky and Steph.

I thought back to June, and the what-ifs ran through my mind. What the doctor said that morning and the way he said it made me believe he felt truly sorry for his failure to diagnose the cancer or to order a biopsy back in June.

"I wish we would have caught it earlier," he said.

I wish we would have too.

Little more than twenty-four hours after my mastectomy, Dr. Connally released me from the hospital. I was in recovery mode. Now I could go home to convalesce. I waited an hour or so for completion of the discharge paperwork. A nurse gave me a flu shot and whisked me off down the hall in a wheel-chair, with a candy striper escort. I could have walked, but the nurse said I should ride. Hospital policy. That was great. I felt like a king with every-one pampering me.

"Are you cold?"

"Do you need a blanket?"

"Here, put this pillow behind you."

"Careful now."

"Watch your step."

Becky and Stephanie provided valet service. Becky pulled the car close to the hospital entrance while my escort and I waited inside in the warmth. It was February in Oklahoma, and the wind could bite. The teenage escort pushed me out the auto-matic glass doors to the curb.

It felt good to be back outside, out of the hos-pital, even if I had been in there only one day. It seemed longer. Fresh air. Independence. Renewed life.

The candy striper tried to help me out of the wheelchair. But I, as any self-respecting older man would, said I could do it myself. I felt no pain, but I moved gingerly, fearing any sudden movement might change all that and undo the surgeon's handiwork.

Stephanie held the car door open, and I tot-tered aboard. Becky drove us home.

My recovery went well from the get-go. My condition and mobility surprised me. I had mor-phine from the hospital still in my system. I supplemented that with hydrocodone twice a day and ibuprofen as often as I needed. Dr. Connally said my chest would feel tight because of the six-inch incision he had made and how tightly he had to bind the breast cavity back together.

I expected a massive, bulky wad of gauze taped over my wound, but it turned out just the opposite when I looked in the mirror. The patch was neat and not nearly as big as I expected.

I felt comfortable at home, back in my element. I knew where everything was. The refrigerator was well stocked. Nurses weren't trying to poke me in the wrong arm.

The next day, Thursday, Becky and I headed across town to campus and my office. I needed to pick up some papers to grade.

I surprised my students in the newsroom.

"Hey, what are you doing here?"

"I wanted to make sure you guys were on the job."

"But you just had surgery."

"I know. Wanna see my scar?" I teased, reaching to unbutton my shirt.

"Oh, gross! No!"

They all scattered and went back to work, content, I presumed, that I was fine. Becky and I returned home, both looking forward to a restful weekend after a traumatic week.

Becky chauffeured me to school and back the first two weeks after surgery. Nobody wanted me driving on heavy drugs. The third week, I drove my F-150 truck. The stick shift didn't bother me as much as the jarring from a pickup truck ride. I didn't wear a T-shirt because it rubbed the incision. Even without the tee, my other shirts irritated the stitches.

I learned a number of lessons—all clichés, I suppose—during my treatment. Live each day. Life is short. Don't waste time. Praise God. Count your blessings. Tell your wife you love her. Tell her often. Kiss her good night.

Becky's mom, Mary, had died suddenly. Becky didn't have the opportunity to say good-bye or to tell Mary how much she loved her. My first wife had died unexpectedly. I didn't get to say good-bye or to tell her one final time how much I loved her. Becky and I both paid the price in heartache and guilt.

I didn't learn my lesson very well that time. I did with this cancer.

The last words out of my mouth every time I left Becky became "I love you." If I should die before I saw her again, I wanted her to remember those words as my last sentiment. I wanted them to remain embedded in her heart and mind.

I realized on the pre-op table that lesson worked two ways. I was the one at risk that time. I regretted not telling the people closest to me more often that I loved them. When Becky kissed me just before the aide wheeled me off to the operating room, I told her I loved her.

Becky and I were no different from anybody else. Our feelings, no doubt, were natural and common for anyone facing a life-threatening situation. We didn't experience any emotional revelations or learn anything that someone else hadn't already learned. We felt what other people feel. We felt what people who are scared feel.

7
CHEMO ANXIETY

The inconveniences of the surgery recovery kept me occupied while I waited to begin eighteen weeks of chemotherapy. I couldn't move my right arm above my head. I couldn't reach. Even extending my left arm pulled the stitches across my chest. I couldn't lift. I couldn't tie my shoelaces.

Someone had to help me at home and at work. I had to concentrate on what I was doing—tying my tie, for example. Little things that I had done effortlessly before surgery.

As the time for chemotherapy neared—a month after surgery—fear of the unknown had me on edge. I worried that the chemotherapy was going to be worse than the disease. People at work asked me about the upcoming treatment. I felt apprehensive and nervous.

My family had a history of cancer, and doctors suspected that hormone blockers might help prevent a recurrence. Surgery, chemotherapy, radiation, and a hormone blocker: that was the combination treatment plan intended to reduce the chances of recurrence. My chances of recurrence dropped from 25 percent without chemotherapy to 10 percent with chemo.

Powerful cancer drugs produced bad side effects. I had read about them. I imagined every possible side effect: nausea, vomiting, pain, fatigue, mouth and throat sores, taste and smell problems, anemia, infection, blood clotting problems, diarrhea, constipation, dry mouth, nerve and muscle effects, skin and nail problems, loss of hair, sunlight sensitivity, flulike symptoms. I worried about them all.

I sensed a need for more spiritual help. I didn't usually gratuitously ask God into my life, but when I was in trouble, when I did ask, He answered.

I'd needed His help years before in Texas, when I was in my early twenties. I had an uncomfortable time adapting to basic training at Lackland Air Force Base in San Antonio and to that sort of military authoritarianism. I adjusted, but some basic trainees never did.

Air Force TIs, or drill sergeants, always picked a slacker out of the chow line, where airman basics were supposed to stand at attention. The same guy many times became their target. A TI we called the Grey Fox showed up with his squadron at the mess hall. This particular TI enjoyed the power of his job. Every training base, no doubt, had a Grey Fox.

My flight had finished eating breakfast, and we waited for the order to fall into formation outside. One chunky fellow from another flight fidgeted as he stood in the chow line. We watched as the Grey Fox eyed him. TIs already had set the misfit back four weeks. Getting set back meant reassignment to a newer flight, so the airman basic had to repeat two weeks of training.

The misfit had started his training in a squadron ahead of mine. After his first setback, he briefly passed through my flight before his second setback. He received forty-five demerits in one inspection. Most trainees got one or two demerits, if any.

The Grey Fox laughed with his TI buddies and then pounced. He humiliated the misfit, a kid with the intelligence of a goose, for all in the mess hall to see. The spectacle—like a bully kicking a helpless dog—made me sick to my stomach.

I acknowledged the philosophy of discipline in the military, and certainly during wartime. Perhaps the TI's action helped save the misfit down the road.

That discipline, no doubt, helped me throughout my life and through the cancer experience. Military discipline gave me a survival attitude, a suck-it-up mentality, a deal-with-it confidence. When life got tough, I knew I could handle it. The discipline, much like tough love, made me grow up, as it did with so many young people. It made me accept responsibility and do things I didn't necessarily want to do but needed to do. I certainly didn't want poison injected into my body, but I felt it was necessary to combat the cancer.

My attitude, that tough mentality, helped me battle cancer. I had the disease. I couldn't reverse the diagnosis. I was backed into a corner, and the only thing I could do was fight—and pray. And I did.

On Tuesday, March 1, a couple of weeks after surgery, Becky and I met with Dr. Sherri S. Durica, a medical oncologist. Dr. Durica thoroughly explained the chemotherapy treatment procedure and gave us literature from the American Cancer Society and drug companies about breast cancer, chemotherapy, and lymphedema. She scheduled a heart test for me the next Friday, a bone scan the following Friday and chemotherapy the third Friday, during spring break.

The first test checked my heart's condition and pumping capability. It would help the oncologist determine the rate and amount of drugs to use.

The day I went for the test, the tech had trouble getting the electrodes positioned on my body so that my heart rhythm would register on the monitor. I flatlined for a couple of minutes before the machine began working properly.

The trouble reminded me of Muskogee Regional Medical Center's pre-op, a sterile-looking room where patients waited for surgery lined up like steers headed for slaughter. I was there—the

time I had forgotten to take off my socks and underwear—because a kidney stone had lodged in my
ureter. As I lay waiting to go into the operating
room, I watched the heart monitor of an elderly
woman bedded beside me. The monitor blipped
up and down, up and down. Suddenly, the blip
stopped. An alarm sounded, and my eyes widened.

The monitor flatlined, and a nurse came running. The old woman stirred. The nurse gazed at
the monitor a few moments and then slapped the
piece of equipment hard. The blip started working
again, up and down, up and down. I thought I
should pray.

Becky cleaned and weeded the front flower beds
and mowed the yard on Saturday. The lawn
mower started on her first pull. How did she do
that? It never started on my first pull.

We drove to Home Depot and picked up ten
bags of red mulch, a flat of yellow pansies, and a
red geranium. The home improvement store
wasn't having one of its better customer service
days. Becky became upset when we couldn't get
anyone to help load the mulch. I pulled the F-150
truck close to the garden area gate, and she loaded
the bags herself. She fumed.

She counted eight employees, mostly young
boys, standing around "picking their noses," as
she put it. None offered to help. After she had
loaded eight of the ten bags, one young employee
made a mistake. He approached and asked her if
he could help.

"It's a little late now!" Becky bellowed for all customers within earshot to hear. "I've had surgery, my husband's had surgery, and we have to load this stuff ourselves. That's just great!"

She still vented as we headed off to the nursery, where we bought eight bags of pecan hulls at $6.95 each, a $2 savings per bag from the price a year earlier. The reduced price pleased Becky, the ex-banker, and she felt better.

We welcomed the coming of spring. It felt good outside. Becky planted pansies in the front-yard flower beds. I hoed the drainage ditch around the bed, and the motion pulled at my stitches. I quickly learned to use my wrists rather than my arms and shoulders. My muscles limbered up, and I surprised myself at how much I could do. We sprinkled pecan hulls on the backyard flower beds and spread mulch, until we ran out, along the pathways.

Becky returned to Home Depot, either forgetting or forgiving past sins of the nose pickers, and bought another ten bags of mulch. She again loaded them herself.

As I started to get out of bed the next morning, the room whirled, much like my December episode of dizziness. I lay down for a few minutes, and the unsteadiness subsided. I ate a sausage biscuit and some Girl Scout cookies and drank a glass of SunnyD and a Mountain Dew, assuming that food and caffeine would lessen the vertigo. I couldn't figure out the problem. I'd gotten plenty of sleep the night before. Maybe I'd overdone the yard work.

The dizziness recurred that evening. I feared it had something to do with the cancer—a brain tumor, perhaps. Doctors never tested for that—or did they? If I could have a breast tumor, why couldn't I have a brain tumor? I hadn't taken any medicine other than painkillers for the cancer and surgery. I worried.

My head swirled and the room turned round and round as I climbed into bed. Becky assured me I didn't have a brain tumor. She said I probably had an inner ear infection.

Aha! An inner ear infection. Why didn't I think of that? An inner ear infection. I can deal with that. I went to sleep.

Dr. Lindsey checked out my ear. He said I didn't have a brain tumor. It was an inner ear infection.

I got word from the Tennessee lawyer that the probate court had ruled I could close my late sister's estate and receive the accountant's fee. That ruling ended years of escalating frustration and stress in handling my sister's affairs as power of attorney. Complications had begun five years earlier when her credit cards were stolen. The Tennessee branch bank's mishandling of the matter eventually resulted in a collection agency hounding me almost daily for three months over an $88 dispute. I refused to pay for the bank's error.

Exasperated after more than a year of haggling, I searched the Internet for the Tennessee and federal banking commissions to file a formal complaint. I wrote to them, insisting that what the bank had done was illegal. The federal agency said it wasn't. I didn't want the expense of suing over $88. I wrote to the national bank's president and CEO and to its board chairman. The CEO responded, apologizing for the bank's mistake and assuring me that a false credit report filed against my sister would be rescinded.

As my sister's health failed, I was dealing long-distance with hospitals, doctors, her assisted-living residence, ambulance services, and insurance companies. After she died and her estate went to probate, I was dealing long-distance with a lawyer, a bonding company, the court clerk, the judge, investment firms, and heirs to the estate.

My sister had $40,000 invested with a charitable institution. The foundation mistakenly thought she had donated the money years earlier. My sister had actually donated the interest, not the principal. When I tried to redeem the principal, I ran into a roadblock with the foundation's lawyer before the matter was settled.

The probate judge's questioning of the accountant's fee had been the proverbial straw that broke the camel's back. I'd become impatient, agitated, and tired of dealing with the delays and frustrations. The case had reaffirmed my belief, formed over years as a journalist, that the judicial system needed serious reform.

Abby, our dog, and I walked our two and a half miles a couple of weeks before chemotherapy was to begin. We set out for the short walk to the

Brookhaven Village Shopping Center. Nice weather, brilliant sun, and not many people out. Perfect. We went farther.

We trekked east down Robinson Street, across the Hollywood movie theater parking lot, past Holiday Inn and Outback Steakhouse, and down the Interstate 35 access road to Sooner Mall.

We walked past Brookhaven Square, where construction on the condominium townhouse addition had spread east toward the interstate. Norman, like most suburbs, had grown rapidly. The city had more than 100,000 residents. The University of Oklahoma added another 26,000 students to the population.

As out of shape as I, Abby was the one panting. I felt surprisingly well.

A week before chemo was to begin, I was at Bill the barber's when he opened up at 8:30 A.M. I wanted a military-style haircut and explained my desire to beat chemo to the punch. I worried about how my head was going to look once all my hair fell out.

Bill said he would leave a little hair, not quite a military cut. He thought it would look better. If I decided later that I needed more hair cut off, he would do it for free. Where else in America but Bill's Barber Shop offered such service?

He asked how I found the tumor. I told him.

The buzz haircut didn't look bad. I went by the newspaper office, and Stacy, the business manager, didn't recognize me. Once she did, she said the new do looked sexy. What can I say?

Becky liked the cut when I got home. She said it took ten years off me. She called me "Colonel."

We shopped Wal-Mart, Ross Dress for Less, and Home Depot. My lack of self-consciousness about my hair surprised me. We bought a thermometer so I could take my temperature every day once chemo started. Becky already had gotten a nonalcoholic mouthwash, necessary in case of mouth sores during treatment.

We traveled north to Stein Mart in Oklahoma City later to look at clothes. Becky's frustration over our month-long ordeal was catching up with her—and me. I offered too much help, and she snapped that she wished she could just look by herself.

I always invaded her space too much. I used to smother her. We'd even had premarriage counseling with the minister. He told me to give Becky her space. I backed off, sort of. I stopped going to her house so often and asking her out every other night. But I began calling her on the phone more frequently. In my eyes, she was simply too hot to leave alone.

That day at Stein Mart, she was just edgy and depressed because of my situation, her hand hurting, trying to stop smoking, taking on a new job, and some of her clothes not fitting anymore.

The incident hurt my feelings too. I was ready to get on with the treatment. We'd had enough anxiety and apprehension, enough fretting about the unknown. I wanted to get it over with.

8

CHEMO SOCKS ME

The doorbell rang.

"Stephanie's here," I yelled.

Becky was still primping in the bathroom.

Steph had come from Edmond, a forty-minute drive. She stopped by our house to ride with us to the medical oncologist's clinic for my first chemotherapy treatment.

Our thoughtful daughter brought a brightly colored gift bag with her. A greeting card stuck out the top of the bag. Beneath the card and a crumpled mass of tissue, I discovered a three-by-five-inch book. *Jesus Calling* was a compilation of devotionals for every day of the year by missionary Sarah Young.

I opened the cover and found a note on the first page: "For Mom and Jack. To help you have good days! I love you. Steph."

A monarch and a frog perched on a leaf faced each other in a color photo on the front of the card. "When face to face with the unexpected, wing it," the message read.

Anxiety about how I might react to my first treatment already had me on edge. Steph's hand-written words inside the card sent my fragile emotions into teary-eyed mode.

> If we knew why, we wouldn't understand.
> If we keep asking why, we'll drive ourselves nuts (And we're already too close to that).
> Keep the faith, a positive attitude and trust in God.
> Oh, and let others do for you (they owe you)—me, especially.
> I love you more than words can say.

Becky hurried out of the bedroom.

"I'm ready. Let's go."

The three of us headed off to the Cancer Care Associates building on the east side of town. My appointment was for 9:30 A.M. It was Friday, March 18.

Becky and I had gone to the same building, a quarter mile past the hospital, the day before. I had to have my blood tested prior to each chemo session. One of the hospital's branch labs was located directly across the hall from my medical oncologist's clinic.

As we entered the lab, two women were coming out. One of them, a cancer victim, I assumed, looked like she was having such a tough day. She appeared to be in her forties or early fifties. She was gaunt, no doubt a skeleton of the woman she once was. She wore no makeup or lipstick, leaving her complexion with an ashen, ghostly hue. Her face was drawn, her eyes hollow and lifeless. She looked right through me. Her hair was disheveled and thinning. Her shoulders slumped, and she shuffled as she walked. Her clothes hung on her. The image of her, so sad and sick, struck me. I felt such heartache and sympathy for her. I wondered if that's how I would look once I began taking chemo treatments.

Only a couple of clients sat in the lab's waiting room. After I checked in at the receptionist's station, we took seats facing a TV fastened high on the wall.

The lab was lined on one side with narrow rows of chairs, back-to-back in front of the TV. If the seats were all filled, half the people would have to listen to the TV, while the other half watched. Administrative cubicles angled down an inner hallway on the opposite side of the room. Before I could have my blood tested, I had to take care of paperwork at one of the cubicle openings.

Becky and I had sat across the counter from a woman as she asked me questions and typed the answers into a computer. Age? Date of birth? Insurance? Primary or secondary? Medications? Spouse's name? By the time we finished, the woman had a permanent record of my identity: my phone number, my beneficiaries, my diseases, my allergies, my blood type, my everything. After each test, she was going to add my blood platelet counts, my white cell counts, my red cell counts. She would know more about me than I knew about myself.

I had to keep digging in my wallet for more cards. The counter quickly became a clutter of insurance cards and forms, consent-to-treat forms, identification cards, medical history forms, and privacy forms.

I had felt relieved to finally go into a small room at the back of the lab. I held out my left arm and let the nurse stick me with a needle and draw blood.

Becky and Stephanie scouted out available seating in the Cancer Care Associates waiting room while I checked in with the receptionist.

"Hello," the receptionist said. "Do you have an appointment?"

"Yes, for 9:30."

"Oh, yes. Mr. Willis."

Cancer brochures lined the countertop in front of the glass window panel that separated the receptionist's area from the waiting room. Guardian angel pins priced at $6 apiece and business cards from each oncologist at the clinic were available on the counter. An empty wheelchair sat off to my left in front of an honor-system bookcase half filled with books on chemotherapy, healing, and other cancer issues. A flyer on a bulletin board promoted a Norman Regional Hospital cancer support group that met the third Tuesday of each month.

A wooden door with a narrow peekaboo slit of a window led to the business office, examination rooms, and the chemotherapy treatment area adjoining the reception area. The waiting room extended off to the right toward a window, providing a view of the parking lot.

The receptionist handed me a clipboard with a ton of forms.

"Please fill these out," she said. "Bring them back to me when you're done."

"Okay."

I turned toward the waiting area to look for Becky and Stephanie.

"You can pay the $25 co-pay now if you'd like," the receptionist said.

"Oh," I stammered. "Okay."

She caught me by surprise. I put the clipboard full of forms on the counter, pulled out my billfold, and passed her a check card. This place wasn't like Wal-Mart, where you paid on the way out.

Becky and Stephanie occupied the first seating cluster, closest to the wooden door. I sat down beside Becky, facing Stephanie, and started filling out the forms.

Two chairs sat on each side of a wooden coffee table. A flat, vertical fountain, three feet tall, was attached to the wall above the table. A nice touch, I thought. But the fountain didn't have any water in it. The rustic ornament probably spattered water, and they had to turn it off. Or perhaps the pump quit working.

An alcove a few feet beyond the fountain contained a display of brochures about breast cancer awareness, FAQs, cancer resources, and wigs and turbans. A poster reminded patients to get their flu shots.

Steph was busy trying to figure out which one of an elderly couple sitting across from us had cancer.

Ten people sat in little groups, congregated by family, I assumed. No one seemed to be there alone. The people seemed ordinary, just like us. No one looked sick, but I knew some of them were. Some thumbed through magazines. Others sat silently staring at the wall. Still others talked among themselves.

The atmosphere seemed different, not like the usual doctor's office. Things looked the same at first glance, but the feeling I had was different. I felt instant empathy when I looked up from my forms and focused on those people waiting to see the doctor or to take their chemo treatment. They didn't have a cold or the flu or a broken arm. They had cancer.

As I watched them, I thought of the statistics I had read earlier. Sixty percent of breast cancer victims lived beyond five years of their diagnosis. That meant that if all of these people had breast cancer, four of the ten sitting there beside us would die from the disease within five years.

Becky and Stephanie were nervous, as I was. This was a new and scary experience.

"Mr. Willis?"

A nurse stepped out from behind the wooden door.

"Would you come back here, please?"

The nurse escorted us to the financial officer's office and introduced us. Becky, Steph, and I met with the woman for fifteen minutes. The woman explained the clinic's financial policies and procedures and what we could expect with billing, payments, and insurance.

Becky had a question.

"How much does one chemo treatment cost?" she asked. "I'm just curious."

We didn't have any idea whether we were looking at hundreds or thousands of dollars. The financial officer wouldn't give Becky a straight answer.

"Oh, don't worry about it," the woman said. "Insurance will take care of it. You've already met your deductible."

"But can you give me an estimate so I can have an idea?"

"You'll only have to pay the $25 co-pay each time you come in."

The woman changed the subject.

We had met our $2,000 deductible fifteen days into my ordeal. That didn't include $1,260 in co-pays and pharmaceuticals the insurance didn't cover. And I hadn't even started chemotherapy.

If this had happened to Becky a year earlier, we would have gone bankrupt. She didn't have medical insurance. The dog crushing her fingers cost us more than $12,000 out of pocket.

We followed a nurse into the treatment room. The place looked harmless enough, but I knew what went on there. I wasn't looking forward to it. Cancer patients, mostly men and women in their fifties and older, sat in recliners with IVs sticking in their arms. Some were relaxed with their eyes closed, as if they were asleep. Others read a book or a magazine. Still others talked with a friend or relative who had come with them.

I felt chilled. Becky and Steph shivered even more. The room was cold.

The room accommodated about eight recliners with IV stands positioned next to them. The recliners, lining the wall in front of the windows, faced a nurses' station half the length of the room. The chest-high barrier around the station reminded me of a long fast-food counter where you order at one end and pick up at the other. Nurses went about their business behind the counter while also monitoring the patients.

A jigsaw puzzle cluttered a table in front of a supervisor's office at one end of the room. A variety of colorful caps and hats, free for the taking, decorated a tall rack standing next to the office door. An assortment of soft drinks, coffee, hot chocolate, juices, and soup sat on a wall counter.

I sat down in a recliner directly in front of the entryway. Becky and Stephanie pulled up chairs in front of me. They began scoping out the other patients while we waited for the nurse. Some patients had come from Ardmore and Ada, small towns south of Norman.

Becky's observations reminded me of a time before we married. I took her to dinner at a restaurant on Lake Fort Gibson, near Muskogee. I sweet-talked and romanced her as we dined. All the while, she looked past me and watched a dispute between the restaurant manager and the people at the table behind me. I knew then she'd missed her calling as a reporter.

Stephanie talked to a cute little woman who wandered in and sat down next to me. She didn't sit long. She was antsy. She half stood up and reached for a handful of caramels, available at each recliner.

"I have a sweet tooth," she told Stephanie.

Stephanie laughed. "All of mine are sweet."

The woman leaned back in her recliner. It was her turn for treatment.

A woman at the far end of the room attracted Stephanie's attention. She was having trouble with her treatment. She was sick. Her recliner was turned to face the window, away from the view of nurses and other patients.

A man and woman who appeared to be her husband and daughter tried to comfort her. The daughter had a cloth in her hand and was wiping her mother's face.

"I felt scared when I saw that woman who was sick," Stephanie later told me. "I prayed for God to not let you get that sick."

"I won't get sick," I said. "Don't worry."

"I don't know what I would do if you did."

I didn't feel any difference in my body chemistry as the nurse affixed an IV to my wrist and the saline began to drip. The first drug helped prevent nausea. The nursing supervisor, Callie, said the chemotherapy drugs included Cytoxan, Adriamycin, and 5-FU, all strong drugs. The Cytoxan dripped forever. Callie injected the other two drugs in ten minutes. The process lasted two hours.

I drank a small Coke because liquids help. As the Cytoxan began dripping, I became chilled again. The nurse said the refrigerated drug cooled my body temperature. She gave me a blanket, and I drank hot chocolate, which warmed me. Actually, I burned my tongue.

Callie said I could eat anything I wanted, but by the fourth treatment, drugs likely would affect my taste buds. I might like things I usually didn't like, and I might dislike foods I usually liked. She said to drink plenty of liquids, no matter what kind, and to vary them.

I could take any prescription medicine. I wasn't to overdo ibuprofen. She recommended Tylenol. Ibuprofen tends to thin blood, as do the chemo drugs that lower the white blood cell count.

Becky asked about sexual activity. Callie said not to get too fatigued or excited. I asked her if she meant Becky or me. The idea of sex made Becky apprehensive, because my body was going to expel the chemotherapy toxins through bodily fluids. We decided to forgo the fun for a while.

The nurse rattled off a list of dos, don'ts, and FYIs:

- Flush the toilet twice for the first forty-eight hours after a treatment.

- If your temperature climbs above 100.5 degrees, call the doctor immediately.
- Your hair might begin to thin after this treatment, but it will come out after the second treatment.
- Eat ice while one of the final two drugs is administered; it helps keep the veins in your mouth cold. That causes them to contract and not receive so much of the drug, which helps prevent mouth sores.
- Wash your mouth with saltwater or non-alcoholic mouthwash three to five times a day to help prevent the ulcers.
- Your white blood cell count will drop to its lowest level ten to fifteen days after the treatment. That's when your immune system will be at its weakest. Then, the cells begin replenishing themselves.

"Are you okay?" Stephanie asked as we left the building. "You look pale."

"I'm fine," I said.

"It's normal," Becky said. "He's supposed to be pale. It goes away."

Stephanie made Becky and I laugh when we got back in the car. She said that during the meeting with the financial officer, she thought: "Oh, my God. How will you all ever afford to pay for this?" She said she considered giving us some money to help pay the bills, but that would have been rude. Instead, she paid for lunch at Taco Bell on our way home.

Becky and I never quite figured out Steph's logic on that one.

Only two good things came out of the first chemotherapy session: It made me quit thinking about the six-inch incision across what used to be my right breast, and I only had five sessions left.

The nightmarish aftereffects shocked my system like nothing I had ever experienced. For the next five days, I lived in my own personal hell, and it affected everyone around me.

Day 1, Saturday, March 29, the day after my first chemo treatment. I remember it well. I woke up in good spirits, and with plenty of energy—I thought. I ate a big breakfast—scrambled eggs, a hash-brown patty, toast, bacon, and a tall glass of SunnyD. I ate it all. Big mistake.

I dusted and vacuumed the sunroom for fifteen minutes, and then I began to feel weak. I usually cleaned the entire house without tiring. A bad taste, triggered by the bacon, filled my mouth. Becky handed me some jellybeans. I rested in the sunroom while she cleaned the house.

I felt guilty that Becky had to do all the work and I wasn't doing my share. I found it difficult to laze around and watch her clean, cook, wash, take care of the finances (she is the ex-banker, remember), and still have to baby me. She had pulled extra duty for a month, picking up the slack while I convalesced from surgery.

I thought I should water the plants outside. Becky said we needed to buy sunscreen for me first. I worked a crossword and watched Abby play. I ate a bowl of chicken noodle soup for lunch while Becky got ready to go to Wal-Mart.

Without warning, my emotions exploded. Despair, no doubt the result of chemo and a month of pent-up anxiety and frustration, engulfed me as I sat at the kitchen table. My life was changing in ways I didn't want it to change. Depression and desperation swept over me—I couldn't work in the yard when I wanted to, I didn't feel I should go with Becky to Wal-Mart and shop around a lot of people, I worried about working with students at school as my white blood cell count decreased and my immune system evaporated, yet I couldn't stay away from them and still do my job. I couldn't control my emotions and started to cry, not knowing whether I wanted to go to Wal-Mart with Becky or stay at home. I doubted the supercenter had that effect on anybody else.

I feared working out on the elliptical machine or the Total Gym because it might affect my recovery. Actually, exercise was helpful during chemotherapy. I had slugged through the winter with plans of getting back in shape in early spring. I was afraid my future was ruined and my life would never return to normal.

Day 2, Sunday, March 20, didn't get any better. I went to sleep fairly quickly the night before but woke up at 1 A.M., then again at 2, restless and unrested. I felt queasy, so I lay there in the middle of the night trying to decide whether to take another nausea pill. Drugs already had taken control of me.

The nurse said I should take the pill at the first sign of nausea. Well past the first sign, I took the extra medication at 3 A.M., not realizing that the pill, dexamethasone, was a steroid. The anti-inflammatory drug helps offset chemotherapy's side effects. It can cause hypertension and psychiatric disturbances such as euphoria and irritability. Side effects of prochlorperazine, the antinausea pill I was taking, included involuntary muscle spasms, tremors, dizziness, jitteriness, constipation, and dry mouth, among others.

I began to cry and I couldn't stop. I needed to go to sleep so I could go to work at noon Sunday. Thinking about work didn't make me go back to sleep. Thinking about my fantasies didn't help. Nothing worked.

I lay there wide-eyed and began to think about a different time in a different life. My mind dwelled on one of the darker periods of my life forty years earlier.

Psychiatrists had diagnosed my first wife, Sandra, with schizophrenia at age twenty-three, six months after we married in 1965. I was twenty-four. Twenty years later, she drowned in the middle of the night, alone, after apparently standing at attention for hours on a rock cliff high above Lake Tenkiller, in eastern Oklahoma. Eventually, she fell into the fifty-foot-deep water and couldn't get out. Sheriff's deputies found witnesses who heard one long, wailing scream from a woman on that June night. Witnesses thought someone had partied too much. Lake patrolmen dragged the water and found Sandra's body two days later.

I had come home from working late at the newspaper at 2 A.M. and found her missing. Witnesses reported seeing her car heading toward the lake that afternoon. She had missed an appointment with her psychiatrist. The two of us, high school sweethearts, had spent many happy days at Tenkiller State Park.

The demons came into Sandra's life shortly after we married. Her psychiatrist told me that schizophrenia often manifests itself with young women about that age. In one instance, Sandra's tormentors ordered her to burn our house. She resisted their demands that time and built a fire in the fireplace on a hot, summer day instead. They would order her to stand at attention for hours at a time while I worked at the newspaper. I would come home and find her drenched in sweat, standing as rigid and straight as a board, her legs, arms, and head locked into position. I would ask her what she was doing, and she would say, "They told me to stand at attention." I would ask who told her to do that. "The people under the ground," she said.

The demons would tell her to jump out of the car while traveling seventy miles per hour down the highway. She would open the passenger car door at a moment's notice and try to jump out. I would frantically grab anything I could—her shirt, her arm—until I could get the car stopped.

I loved and adored her so much. Her condition almost drove me insane too.

The Oklahoma State Medical Examiner's Office ruled the death a suicide, something I refused to accept over the years. Suicide wasn't in Sandra's nature, and it was practically impossible for someone to commit suicide by drowning. I was furious at the medical examiner. How could he possibly know what was in her mind high on that cliff that night? Who was he to proclaim she committed suicide? He was guessing, putting two and two together, making an assumption, dealing with a probability. My brother told me to let it go, that it didn't matter anymore because Sandra was at peace and in a better place.

Over the years, I found myself rethinking the medical examiner's finding and what my brother said. I could never let go of the thought that Sandra might have ended her life. I didn't believe she had. At least now I understood how she could have contemplated that act.

Reflection over time and seeing what drugs do to a person physically and emotionally, feeling the effects of depression and the uncertainty of a potentially deadly disease, gave me a different perspective. I could see how someone without hope of getting better, someone who lived for twenty years with despair, could contemplate suicide.

I realized why Sandra had sometimes refused to take her medication, even though the primitive drugs at that time did make her more sociable. I understood how more than twenty years of drugs and mental illness could become too much for her to bear. I realized I wanted her, her life with me, for my sake and not for her sake.

As I lay there remembering, I could accept her death as a suicide more easily than I could in 1985 when the medical examiner ruled her drowning a suicide. If I felt so devastated after one chemotherapy treatment, how terrible must she have felt all those years? I didn't understand how she had endured her agony and the demons in her mind for so long.

My mind and education told me how these cancer drugs could benefit me, but my instincts, much like an animal's, I suspect, told me just the opposite. The drugs took away control of my chemistry and my body's natural system. I wondered what crazy SOB came up with the idea that to kill bad cancer cells, you had to kill good white blood cells that combat infection. Even in nature, the strongest survived by killing the weakest, not by killing the strongest. We put ladybugs in the garden to kill pests that damaged the plants. The ladybugs didn't destroy the garden in the process of trying to save it.

We were killing the strongest cells, the fighters, and it devastated me. Even though I knew science to date had proved that this treatment worked, I still cursed my oncologist that night for poisoning me.

I had always been sensitive to drugs, and these overwhelmed me. I had to believe the reaction would get better once my body adjusted.

My late sister from Tennessee had taken twenty-one pills a day preceding her death from Parkinson's disease: pills to counteract pills, medicine to counteract medicine, to control her life, to disrupt the natural flow and order of her body.

My sister Inabelle didn't want to take pills to help her eighty-three-year-old memory, because she'd had an adverse reaction to them earlier. I understood now.

Becky, like her dad in so many ways, never liked to take drugs—no aspirin, no cold medicine, no Tums, no nothing. I understood now.

Medicine changed the way we lived and improved our lives. It allowed people who might have died earlier to have more longevity, worth, and dignity. But drugs didn't cure; they only treated symptoms. Sometimes they caused more complications than they solved. I had to believe that in the long run it was God's plan and not just man's ego at work.

I cried that morning at the least little thing. I felt better after I went to work, but I got tired quickly and was so emotional I went home early. I went to bed and slept twelve hours.

Day 3, Monday, March 21, an uneventful day. The twelve-hour rest helped. I ate scrambled eggs and toast with grape jelly for breakfast. I went to campus late. Acid indigestion set in. I chewed Tums two and three at a time. I worked until after 5:30 and didn't notice feeling fatigued until I plopped on the couch at home. I took a Tagamet, ate two fish fillets and a baked potato, and went to bed.

Day 4, Tuesday, March 22. My emotional state seemed better. I ate tuna fish with my eggs and toast with some aftertaste. I told Becky my mouth tasted like I had a chunk of defecation stuck in my upper throat.

Nonalcoholic mouthwash helped. I went to work late again, making my workday much shorter.

My pee thickened as if I needed to drink more liquids. I passed gas frequently, and the smell ran me out of my chair at times. Drugs didn't mix well with eggs and tuna fish. I dined on chicken noodle soup for lunch. No sweets or desserts. I had no desire for the Sno Ball or chocolate-covered Dipp I packed with lunch most days. The banana still didn't look good. Throughout the day, I snacked on hard candy and caramels to keep my mouth moist.

I didn't go to bed as early that night, but when I did, I couldn't sleep. I kept thinking of Del Monte's diced peaches. I never got up to satisfy the dry-mouth symptoms.

Constipation set in. My stomach began to hurt. I got up and took a stool softener, hoping my bowels would loosen up. They didn't. I hurt through the night and dozed, not sleeping any longer than an hour at a time. Nothing helped.

Day 5, Wednesday, March 23, the day I remembered most, my longest and hardest. I didn't feel like getting up at 8 o'clock, two hours later than I usually got up, but I did. The smell of toast and eggs cooking in the kitchen turned my stomach as I came out of the bedroom. I ate them anyway. I felt queasy, and my hands trembled. I lay down on the recliner and stayed quiet to ease my discomfort.

I arrived at work, dragging. A couple of times, I thought I would go home, but I had scheduled an alumna to speak with our students. I wanted to see Jennifer Johnson, who was working for the Wall Street Journal Online in New York. She had become so successful so fast, just two years out of college. I couldn't wait to see our students' reaction to her.

I took a nausea pill late that afternoon, and it helped. I should have taken more throughout the week. Earlier in the week, I stopped taking the pill three days after chemo, just as the nurse had instructed. That was too soon.

It seemed odd that the Campbell's classic chicken noodle soup I took for lunch every day still tasted good. I used caramels to get the aftertaste out of my mouth. Water tasted better. Soft drinks didn't.

I never lost my appetite, though. I expect that was how I maintained my muscle definition. Whatever my body called for, I ate. I must have added a million dollars to the bottom line for KFC, Church's Chicken, and Tyson Foods.

Day 6. At 4:30 P.M. on the dot, the phone rang at work.

"Hi. How're you feeling?" Becky asked.

"Hey. What's going on? Are you at work?"

"Yes. It's really slow today. I was just checking to see how you were doing."

"I've been busy, and I hadn't thought about it, but, you know, all of a sudden I feel pretty good."

"That's good."

"Wow, now that I think about it, I feel real good."

I was experiencing some kind of a breakthrough. I didn't know whether it was Becky's call or perhaps anticipating two days off for the weekend, or that the drugs had finally flushed out of my system. For the first time in a week, I seemed normal, like the relief you feel when you wake up and the fever from a cold or the flu has broken during the night. I felt as if armies of endorphins, those tiny substances that form within us to relieve pain, had come to rescue me.

I didn't have much energy. But I had hope now that every day during this eighteen-week ordeal didn't necessarily mean having to go through the hell of the past five days. Depression had crept in and socked me hard a time or two. I adapted the old sports adage—take it one game at a time. I took it one day at a time. I saw a ray of normalcy during chemotherapy.

When Becky called me at work, it was such a welcome surprise. Both of us had always understood that the workplace was not for personal business. We rarely took personal phone calls at work. Becky used to threaten Stephanie when she was growing up: "If you're not dying, or it's not an emergency, don't call us at work."

Becky had made an exception, and I was pleased. Just hearing her voice soothed me and made me feel loved and not so alone. I felt vulnerable and down much of the time. Nausea was just a thought away. During the entire ordeal, I felt reclusive. I knew the cancer was my battle. I felt that no one but God could really help me get through each day. I knew Becky and Stephanie would have traded places with me and taken my pain. I knew how much they loved me. Still, it was my fight. The drugs' side effects weren't making it easier. They made me extremely emotional. A sympathetic voice did wonders for me.

Becky began to check on me every afternoon. I could stick the phone to my ear, glaze over for the moment, and go into our little world where I felt safe and protected. She was just calling to see if there was anything she could do or get for me that would make me feel better. She said she just wanted me to know how much she loved me.

I worried how every little ache and pain might affect me. Callie, the nursing supervisor, had said some patients tended to blame everything on the chemo. If my vertigo had happened after the treatments began, I likely would have blamed it on the chemo too. When I sneezed, I felt like I was getting a cold. When I woke up with a dry throat, Becky had to remind me about postnasal drip. When my stomach got upset, I figured it was a virus. Becky said it was acid indigestion. During flu season when my body ached, I thought I was catching the flu.

When our dog, Abby, had a choking episode, I felt as if I had the same thing. I coughed and choked. Dr. Lindsey laughed when I told him I might have what the dog had.

After the first chemo session, I gave the dog some of the ice from my glass, and she threw up. I wondered if I had left chemo juices on the ice. I figured it had happened too fast for that and the cancer treatment had antivomit stuff in it anyway. I suspected the dog had a virus—or acid indigestion.

That night, I ate chicken and rice. As the night wore on, a putrid metallic taste filled my mouth and my teeth began to ache. I took two ibuprofen tablets to stop my teeth from aching and for the dull headache that resulted.

Thinking about the chemo drugs stopped me from thinking about the irritation in my breast, though. The surgery wound got better each day.

Two weeks after the first session, things were looking up at Jack and Becky's house. I walked three miles on the elliptical machine and grunted through twenty sit-ups, twenty over-the-head pulls, and twenty arm curls on the Total Gym. That was my most strenuous exercise since I had surgery. I felt my strength coming back.

I worked outside for the first time since chemo began. I wore a long-sleeved shirt, gloves, and an old Boy Scout wide-brimmed hat to shade the bright morning sun.

A hundred tulips—reds, yellows, and purples —stood on tiptoe, reaching for the sun. Blossoms three inches in diameter exploded with vibrant color on the flowerbed mounds along the winding, dry creek bed. Most of the daffodils still bloomed. The blades from Dutch iris and daylilies poked skyward, and two white crabapple trees flourished above them all. The sand cherry's pink buds complemented the crabapples.

Even though I hadn't lost that much hair yet, the sun still felt hot on my head. I dreaded the Oklahoma summer already.

9

I CAN DO THIS

The alarm went off at 6 A.M., and I scrambled to quash it. I lay there listening to the mockingbird perched atop our house, singing for the neighborhood. I thanked God for my many blessings.

I had tried to thank Him for my life, my family, and our loved ones every single morning since I'd heard Kathie Lee Gifford on *Live with Regis and Kathie Lee* years ago. I usually didn't watch the show, because I was at work, but for some reason I was watching that particular day. Kathie Lee said she thanked the Lord every morning for the day, and that struck me. I thought I should do the same thing.

I prayed often enough, I thought, and I knew the Lord's Prayer and its daily message, but for some reason I didn't make a point to thank God every single day. I didn't thank Him for my simplest and most basic blessing—each day He allowed me to wake up and live my life.

Kathie Lee's words that day changed me. I realized I needed to be conscious of God every day, every moment if possible. I needed to be more mindful of the source of my simplest blessings. I needed to praise Him every day and not get so wrapped up in day-to-day living that I ignored Him or took Him for granted. It was that feeling you got with a New Year's resolution. You rededicated yourself. But I realized I couldn't dismiss prayer and divine gratitude after a couple of months like I dismissed a resolution to exercise more. I had to recommit myself to include God in everything, all the time.

I knew I couldn't make it through this illness by myself. I needed God.

I believed that when all of us faced trouble, especially life-threatening trouble, we grasped for spirituality, some power greater than ourselves. Those situations made us realize our mortality. They strengthened or rekindled any religious upbringing we may have had, or they prompted a search for a safe haven if we didn't have that spiritual grounding. We held on tighter to whatever or whomever we believed in. To fight cancer, I thought it was even more important that I thanked God every day.

When I talked to God, I felt close to Him. I knew I wouldn't be here except for Him. I prayed for strength, courage, guidance, and wisdom. I asked Him to forgive my sins. I felt Him beside me, and I knew I could tackle anything.

I was nervous about the second treatment after my less-than-stellar performance the first go-round three weeks earlier. As the April 8 appointment neared, I became more anxious. I didn't look forward to the remaining five sessions. At least I knew what to expect this round, though.

I had my blood tested at the cancer lab. The test registered my hemoglobin, platelets, white blood cell count, red blood cell count, and numerous other factors. That allowed chemo nurses to determine if I had anemia or any inflammation or infection and to judge how well I could fight infection.

If my white blood cell count was low, it meant my body was too weak to receive another dose of chemo drugs and could put me at risk for severe infection and interrupt my chemo treatments. I passed the test, so I was a go for my second session later that day.

Oklahoma's spring clouds rolled overhead and it looked like rain as Becky and I headed for the chemo appointment with Dr. Durica.

I worried about the drug buildup in my body over time. I asked the nurse at the weigh-in and vitals check if this second session and future sessions would cause a buildup and make me sicker.

She half smiled and looked at me, but she didn't say anything. Her eyes told me what I wanted to know.

"I've got it," I said, forcing a half smile myself.

I expected that. I presumed the more drugs you put into your body, the longer it took them to dissipate.

"Different people react differently to subsequent chemo sessions," the nurse said. "Some do just fine and others don't."

I didn't know how I would handle it if the second treatment's aftereffects were worse than the first's. After the initial treatment, I felt better each day after the first week. But that first week was a bitch. I expected with each treatment, the recovery period would take longer. I would have to learn to adapt.

Dr. Durica seemed pleased with my progress and how I had reacted to the first chemo treatment. I told her about the tough first week. She said I should take another nausea pill, prochlorperazine, and that might help stop the terrible feeling.

The doctor also gave me a third prescription for nausea. She said if the first two didn't ease my discomfort to take the third one too.

Great.

I rested Friday afternoon after the second treatment, remembering that I didn't take it easy after the first session, and I paid for it. I didn't want that to happen this time.

Saturday went well, with lethargy the only side effect. I took the double dose of nausea medicine Friday night and Saturday, as Dr. Durica had instructed. It helped. I didn't feel nauseous.

I went to bed about 8:30 P.M. but slept in spurts. The medicine caused an overdose-like reaction. I had never experienced an overdose, but I expected this felt like one.

While dozing, flashes of brilliant reds and blues merged with a psychedelic strobe-light effect and flooded my nightmarish state. Japanese-like lanterns with diamond-shaped tinfoil shards twirled and danced in front of me. Two lanterns, one tall and skinny, the other shorter and fatter and off to the right, reflected the strobe lights, turning and twisting the vibrant colors, piercing my closed eyes. The light effect came and went in my mind.

My teeth chattered slightly, not quite like that caused by a chill, but like an uneasiness or nervousness.

Sunday morning, I had absolutely no energy. My hands trembled slightly. I felt weak and strange, that tingly feeling when your system is out of whack and you don't know what's wrong. I didn't have to be at the newspaper until noon, so I lounged on the easy chair and dabbed at the crossword puzzle.

As the afternoon dragged on at work, I developed a weird sensation and my hands began to tremble uncontrollably. I couldn't hold them steady. I couldn't type. I couldn't grade papers. I couldn't write. I couldn't concentrate.

I went upstairs and told my colleague, Kathryn, about my symptoms. She said my medicine could be a steroid and that might cause my hands to tremble. I left work early and went home.

I called Dr. Bill. He confirmed that dexamethasone was a steroid. Great, I had already taken four double-dose sets of the pills. Now I was probably going to die from a steroid overdose. Maybe I should have had my stomach pumped.

I didn't take the steroid Sunday night, and Monday morning I wasn't dead. Actually, aside from the tremors and fatigue, the difference in how I felt after the second session and after the first session bordered on spectacular. I felt great.

My drug debacle reminded me of the 1960s and 1970s. I didn't do drugs or smoke pot back then. I never got into the hippie and flower child phenomenon, though it was popular to say you had if you were from my generation. I wore the flared pants like Sonny and Cher, but I didn't dance the dance.

I guess Merle Haggard was, indeed, singing about me, an editor from Muskogee, with his famous rendition of "Okie from Muskogee":

> We don't smoke marijuana in Muskogee;
> We don't take our trips on LSD.
> We don't burn our draft cards down on Main Street;
> We like livin' right, and bein' free.
>
> I'm proud to be an Okie from Muskogee,
> A place where even squares can have a ball.
> We still wave Old Glory down at the courthouse,
> And white lightnin's still the biggest thrill of all.

The lyrics to that song had rallied support for the war in Vietnam. They represented, at the time, what many people knew were the values and strengths of this country. Muskogee and Oklahoma were either out of touch with reality when the protesting and shooting began or, more likely, years behind the agenda setting of the East and West Coasts.

The strongest drinks I ever had were laced with caffeine—Coke and Pepsi and Mountain Dew—and the strongest drug an aspirin for a headache.

I was a staunch supporter of President Lyndon Johnson and all he stood for at the time. I was solidly in the Johnson and Robert McNamara camp, blaming communism and the domino theory in Southeast Asia and Vietnam as the greatest threat to our American way of life. I condemned the antiwar protesters—at Kent State University and elsewhere.

Age and wisdom, if not youth and courage and outrage, had given me more than one occasion to reflect on a misguided philosophy.

Our government had fed us a line. The Pentagon Papers proved it. Americans lost faith in our government. I lost faith in it. Kennedy had begun to withdraw American troops, but he was assassinated in 1963. Johnson became president and used the Gulf of Tonkin incident in 1964 to escalate American troop levels. Publication of the Pentagon Papers by *The New York Times* revealed how the U.S. government had expanded its involvement in Southeast Asia while Johnson was promising the American people just the opposite. We couldn't get accurate information because the government was censoring the news.

Many Americans believed we were fighting an immoral war. We were interfering in a foreign civil war. We wanted the Saigon government to reform, something it wasn't going to do. We had no plan to win the war. We used a conscription policy that allowed middle-class Americans to avoid the draft. That forced the lower class to fight the war. There were more than enough issues at the time to make me change my mind.

My euphoric reaction to the second chemo session carried through the following weekend. My sleep pattern changed. I began waking up at 4 A.M., feeling rested. My stomach still gurgled and I still belched. Flatulence took over occasionally, but not with the same rank odor I sometimes expelled after session number one.

I couldn't help but be amused at Stephanie. She offered to bring me some beans, a source of protein recommended for cancer patients. I declined the musical fruit she had prepared, even if protein would have been good for me. But thanks anyway.

I suspected that the steroids caused me to wake up so early, with nothing to do in the wee hours. At first, I lay in bed, mulling my plight. All sorts of thoughts ping-ponged around in my brain. I was wasting time lying there. I slipped out of bed, trying not to disturb Becky, pulled on my sweat shorts and fumbled in the dark for my Reeboks. I bumped my head against the wall, trying to tie the shoelaces. My shorts felt funny. They were on backwards. Trying to balance on one leg and then the other, I took the shorts off, found the front, and put them on again. I peeled the Breathe Right tape off my nose, rattled my glasses off the night table, and tiptoed toward the bedroom door.

"Where're you going?" a voice in the dark asked.

"Oh!" I exclaimed. "What are you doing awake?"

"Somebody was making too much noise and woke me up."

The voice didn't sound like one that had been asleep.

"Sorry. Go back to sleep. I'm just going to go get on the computer."

"Are you sure you're okay? Don't you need to sleep?"

"I was just lying there anyway. I thought of something, and I need to write it down. I'll be back to bed in a little while."

I'd done that before. I'd wake up in the middle of the night, start thinking about work, and then have to get up and jot down a brainstorm so I wouldn't forget it by morning.

I pulled the door shut behind me. Becky could go back to sleep. Landscape lights filtering through the front windows lit my way to the computer room, a converted bedroom with a north window facing Bob White Avenue. I flipped on the light.

As I sat down at the computer desk and switched on the PC, I had an idea. I should start keeping a journal. I wished I had kept a journal growing up, but I didn't. Much of my childhood was lost now. A journal would give me something to do at 4 in the morning. A woman at work told me she got up at 3:30 and wrote. She said that was when she did her best work.

I never wrote for pleasure. All of my writing as a journalist related to work. A journal seemed a good idea. It would allow me to document my progress with the cancer treatment. The cancer society literature suggested that keeping a journal would help doctors better monitor my treatment.

Over the next few weeks, I found writing in the journal very personal and therapeutic. I focused on writing, like a hobby, and it took my mind off the cancer and chemotherapy, even if only for a few hours. I could say things in a computer file that I couldn't say to Becky or Stephanie or to anyone else. I could say what I was thinking.

I woke up about 3 o'clock one April morning and felt what I thought was God inside me, cleansing my body. I felt it for a few fleeting seconds, a swift sensation, not an all-night feeling. It came fast, and it went away just as fast. But I felt it clearly. It wasn't a dream.

I read in the cancer literature about people visualizing various things cleansing their bodies. I didn't put a lot of stock in that at the time.

However, I knew you could visualize getting well. I did it once. When I started working at the newspaper in Muskogee in the early seventies, Sandra and I were living in an apartment, new in town, and we didn't have a doctor.

I developed a severe cold and felt as if I could easily die and feel better for it. I couldn't get in to see a doctor. After calling every physician in town, I finally got so mad because none was taking new patients that I willed myself well. I knew I didn't do that all by myself. I prayed. Overnight, I began to feel better, and I went to work the next day feeling fine. It normally took me two weeks, sometimes longer, to get over a cold.

In my mind, I knew my euphoria now was some sort of chemical reaction, probably to the dexamethasone. But in my soul, I knew God was cleansing any remaining cancer and the poisonous drugs from my body—making me whole again—just as He had done that night so long ago in the Muskogee apartment.

Some mornings, depending on my mood, I turned on the CD player and lost myself in the rapture of the music. Sometimes the ballets and the symphonies made me so emotional I couldn't write, and I had to turn them off. But if I chose not to turn them off and let my mind drift, the music carried me away to places where I didn't have any problems or nausea or illness.

One morning, I couldn't seem to turn the music off. Sarah Brightman and "The Phantom of the

Opera" stirred me. I thought of Sandra. The music engulfed me, and I felt Sandra and God close to me. I felt the Lord, as if He were wrapping His presence around me—like a mother wraps her arms around her child—assuring me that I was safe, that I didn't have to worry, and that He would take care of me. I sensed that Sandra was looking down on me too, watching over me, and helping me fight.

I thought of Sandra in that way. I believed in angels, for lack of a better word to call them. I believed in the afterlife and the spirits of the after- life. I believed they—through God—helped us throughout our lives.

Stephanie said that when she prayed for me, she asked for help from Sandra and others who had left this earth: my parents, my sisters, her Me- maw and Pa-paw, and her Nana.

I knew that when my mood was just so and I was stimulated by beautiful music, my mind found a connection with something I loved. I thought of Becky and Stephanie. I thought of San- dra. And I thought of God.

For some reason, I became overly emotional every time I thought about God. I didn't know if I simply couldn't handle my emotions or if there was another reason. I thought of all the blessings He had given me, and I felt overwhelmed with gratitude. I would start crying, and I wouldn't know why.

Abby and I took our favorite walk to Brookhaven Village. Customers scurried around Starbucks and a fitness gym stuck in the corner of the shopping complex. A new business to Norman, Talbots, was scheduled to open in a renovated retail location in late summer. Contractors had made noticeable progress. Becky submitted her application and interviewed with the company. She could work three blocks from our house doing what she loved most, selling clothes.

10
LIVING WITH CHEMO

Changes in my body came in waves after chemo treatments began. Facial hair vacated my body first. Then the hair on my back disappeared, and my arms didn't look quite so hairy. The hair on my head felt like the dormant February Bermuda grass in my front yard: dry, prickly, and crunchy.

While drying off after taking a shower, I felt a bump on my head about an inch above my left ear. It hurt when I rubbed my head with the towel. It felt like a pimple under the skin trying to break out. I started to worry. Maybe it was a tumor. I would wait and see.

The spot hurt again the next day with no sign of a pimple breakthrough. A day later, the pain moved around to the other side of my head. Then the right side hurt and the left side didn't. It wasn't a pimple. Maybe it was a tumor. I worried. Becky said it was my hair follicles irritating my scalp as my hair prepared to fall out.

I worried some more. I asked Dr. Durica, the medical oncologist, about the mystery at my next appointment. She said it was my hair follicles irritating my scalp as my hair prepared to fall out.

I'd always had a lot of hair. It was thick on my head, with patches on my chest, stomach, and below. Becky told me after our first intimate encounter twenty years ago that she liked a man with hair on his chest. I puffed up, knowing I had a lot. When I reminded her of what she had said so long ago, she told me I might have had one or two little hairs on my chest when we got married. She said it was only after we got married that I grew hair on my chest.

I dabbed a little of Becky's greasy hair stuff on my head and I was good for the day, Oklahoma wind and all.

The hair on my head gradually began to thin after treatments began. Then hairs started falling out in record number. I left fine, gray telltale signs wherever I went. My wife tracked me. She knew if I had used the kitchen sink, sat at the dinner table, or lounged in the sunroom or the living room. Hair rained down on my desk at work, in my pickup truck, on my shirt. Becky said I shed more than our dog.

When I lathered my hands and rubbed shampoo over my head in the shower, a mass of gray, dark hair covered my hands. Hair clung to the walls and the shower door and partially hid the drain. I stuck my hands up and out over the shower door and called for Becky.

"Look, I've got Big Foot's hands," I said.

I went back to the barbershop after the second treatment to get a trim for what little hair I still had. Bill the barber wasn't working. His daughter-in-law was cutting hair. I thought, "Oh no, here it comes again—more money." The last time I'd sat in her barber's chair, she looked me over and said I had changed my do. I had made the mistake of letting someone else cut my hair while I was out of town, and I guess the guy made a barber's faux pas. The hair looked whopper-jawed on my head.

When the daughter-in-law had to fix the mistake, she charged me $12 instead of the usual $11. Bill's shop sported a big sign next to a poster of Oklahoma Memorial Stadium: "Haircuts $11." Old-time barbershops that charged $11 for a haircut still existed, but you had to hunt for them.

The daughter-in-law said it took her longer to cut my hair after the other barber butchered it, so she charged me an extra dollar. I hadn't forgotten that.

As I climbed into the chair this time, she asked me if I wanted the number one cut or the number one and a half cut. I didn't know what she meant, and I certainly wasn't going to ask. I assumed the number one was the shortest cut, almost bald, and the other was longer. I took the number one. After she finished, I wanted to see myself in the mirror to make sure I had made the right decision. I had.

"Chemo?" she asked.

"Yep."
"That'll be eleven dollars."

Two days in a row I didn't shave. That didn't feel right. I had shaved nearly every day for fifty years. If I used six blades a month all those years, that meant I'd purchased 3,600 razor blades in my lifetime. The Gillette Company should have given me a plaque.

Shaving came as routinely to me as brushing my teeth and combing my hair. I found myself grazing my fingers across my cheek and chin more often. I could feel baby stubble on my face, much like that of a teenager just beginning to sprout whiskers. The razor didn't meet much resistance, except for the renegade whisker.

Becky asked me one morning why I was shaving. I took that as an insult to my masculinity. I'd always shaved.

The bathroom could be an adventure. My stream had been slowing down and getting funky for several years—old-age prostate. At the least opportune moment, I could dribble all over myself if I wasn't paying attention.

Men understood what I was talking about. It wasn't that we intended to make a mess or miss the stool; we sprayed sometimes, and we certainly weren't going to squat. Squatting was a woman thing.

I wore new pants to school, and I tried not to spray myself, but I did anyway. Think of one of those new garden-hose nozzles with the adjustable settings. I was on the "shower" setting that day. Some days it was the "jet" setting; some days the "flat" choice; and as I got older, the thing could even be on "mist" occasionally. Those pants were a light brownish rust color with a vertical pattern of fine streaks. They were beautiful, but they showed stains. I was being particularly careful.

My diuretic kicked in, and I had been beating a path to the bathroom all day. I dribbled and it sprayed the floor, my shoes, my pants, and my hand. I tried to squeeze the kinks out to steady the stream, and it got worse. All I needed was a student to come into the bathroom and think I was milking the monkey.

I had to rub the pants with a paper towel before the residue dried and stained. A big spot on the professor's pants in front of class wasn't a good thing.

A professor came into the bathroom to do his business, and before he began washing his hands, he cranked the paper towel holder lever two or three times. He washed his hands, tore off the paper, and dried his hands. How strange, I thought. I had never seen that.

With my immune system on the fritz, I began doing the same thing. I cranked out the paper towels, pushed the soap dispenser, washed my hands, tore off the towel, and then dried my hands.

I took it a step further. I used the towel to shut off the faucet and to open the door, and then hoped

I could toss the towel in the trashcan without missing as I scooted out the door.

I woke up Easter morning feeling good. My nose dripped, and I thought, "Oh no, a cold." Becky would say it was just postnasal drip. I took an Allegra-D. For allergies, I usually cut the tablet in half. I took a whole tablet that day.

Gigi and Francie called to say they were on their way to Norman. They didn't come to Norman often. I wondered if they thought I was dying.

On Easter eight years earlier, Becky's mom had sat the three sisters down and told them: "I don't want you to worry. Everything's taken care of, but I want you all to know that I have cancer."

Mary was only seventy-two at the time. She still attended dancing classes and performed in recitals.

"I thought she would be okay," Becky said. "As much as I hate to admit it, I knew very, very little about my mom's cancer."

Becky and Mary were close, but her mother and father were from the old school. They didn't share their problems. Mary rarely talked about her cancer or her treatment. Every time she did, she assured Becky everything was all right.

In May, Becky and I stopped by Frank and Mary's house in Muskogee on our way to Branson. Mary didn't feel up to going with us on vacation. She was about to start her chemotherapy treatment. It was the first time in four years that Mary hadn't gone with us.

In August, we headed back to Branson. Mary thought she should stay home. She didn't have much energy after her chemo treatment began. Becky and I bypassed Muskogee and went up I-44 to Springfield, just north of Branson. We stayed at the same bed-and-breakfast inn on Table Rock Lake where we always stayed with Mary and Becky's sisters. We saw a show that night.

About 6 A.M. Sunday, somebody knocked on our door. The owner of the bed-and-breakfast had a telephone call for us. Francie said Mary was in the hospital and we needed to get back to Muskogee fast. We drove ninety miles per hour and made it to the hospital. Francie was standing outside.

"Mom's gone," she told Becky.

I felt so sorry for Becky as she grieved. She regretted not spending more time with her mom, but she hadn't realized how seriously ill Mary was. Becky felt guilty for not knowing more about cancer.

"I think of my poor mother having to go through that whole ordeal by herself," Becky said. "I wish I would have known better."

Frank couldn't talk about Mary after she died, so Becky never really knew what happened. Frank loved Mary so much he couldn't say her name for the longest time. Becky wouldn't push him for answers.

"We three sisters didn't know about cancer when Mom died," she said. "Once you know what cancer is about, you become more aware. You become a better listener. You become more compassionate."

Six years later, Frank became ill. Becky needed to spend time with him. At eighty-two, Frank didn't have that many years left. Becky had worked constantly except for two weeks of vacation, the only time she could take off and still get paid. She had to make do with day trips—a five-hour round-trip drive—to see him on Saturdays.

Becky talked about quitting her job at Dillard's for a year, but she loved clothes and she loved outfitting her customers. Just before the Christmas season in 2003, Becky quit the job she loved so much and prepared to spend time with her dad. Within two weeks, Frank's health became critical. He suffered in the hospital on Christmas Day, not expected to live. Gigi, between jobs, and Becky moved into the little family home where they'd grown up in Muskogee to take care of their dad when he came home from the hospital. Francie already lived there in an adjoining mother-in-law apartment. Frank died in February.

After I was diagnosed, Becky told me she felt that taking care of Frank and staying with him was God's way of preparing her for my cancer.

Looking back, I realized I might have overreacted to my fear of cancer and chemotherapy. I didn't know enough about cancer or enough to make intelligent decisions or plans.

I thought I wouldn't be able to do much during the spring and summer. That wasn't the case. After I got past the first few days of chemo, the biggest problem I had was fatigue. It was worse than I expected. I had trouble getting my strength back, as if I were in a winter funk. I just couldn't get back to the way I always felt in the spring.

My recurring dizziness worried me. Becky and I were starting out on our morning walk and saw our next-door neighbor Ann, a single woman, trying to trim her yaupon holly tree. The tree was taller than the gutters on her house.

I grabbed our ladder and began to help her trim the tree. The morning was hot and humid. I had climbed the ladder to clip the top branches when I began to feel light-headed and flushed. I lay down on Ann's front porch and tried to clear my head. Ann brought me a glass of cold water. I tried to resume the trimming several times. I lay down again. Becky finally said enough was enough.

She took my arm and began to escort me home. I don't remember much after that. She said I was wobbly, flushed, and talking very slowly. She didn't know if I was having a heatstroke or if this was a symptom of the chemo. She said that all of a sudden I began to collapse. She yelled for Ann to help. I passed out for about thirty seconds. She said it seemed forever. They got me home, cooled me off, and made me stay inside the rest of the day.

Two days later, I got up to use the bathroom around 2 A.M. Becky was awake, but I didn't know it. A couple of minutes later, she heard a bam-bam. She figured I was out of toilet paper and slamming cabinet doors to show my frustration. Then all was quiet. She thought I was just doing my business, and she went back to sleep.

Actually, the bam-bam she heard was my head hitting the wall and then the tile floor. I didn't realize I was falling, but I guess my head hitting the wall jarred me out of my state. Immediately, I saw the floor coming up to meet my face. "Damn, that hurt!" I got up off the floor and went back to bed.

I didn't know whether I'd fallen asleep doing my business or whether I'd fainted. The doctor said that when I urinated, my blood pressure decreased, and I probably just fainted. Becky and I began to monitor my blood pressure morning and night to decide what I could and couldn't do or if I needed additional medication.

Becky worried when I tried to do everything I had done before chemo. On the Fourth of July, she caught me mowing, edging, and trimming trees in the neighbor's yard. The guy was trying to do it, but he didn't have the proper equipment. I went across the street to help him after I finished taking care of our lawn.

Becky reminded me that my system was pretty much shut down. She reminded me that my blood count was low, my blood pressure was low, and I had virtually no immune system.

"Slow down!" she said.

I didn't realize it was 95 degrees outside that day.

11
THE HALFWAY POINT

Every spring, the mockingbird took his station on top of our house about 5 A.M. each morning and began his melodious reveille. I suspected he picked our house because it had the highest roof and he could safely watch the morning's activity unfold below him. Rosy-colored finches accompanied him from their roosts in the photinia and holly bushes along the back fence.

The chimes Becky's dad had made from five two-foot pieces of pipe and fishing line clanged to the beat of Oklahoma's wind gusts beneath the eave. I loved that symphony in the early morning, more this year than the last. Instead of going back to sleep until the alarm went off at 6, I usually lay in bed and listened. My life was changing so fast, I wanted to enjoy every single minute.

The morning of my third chemo treatment was different, though. I woke up in a funk. I could tell it was going to be one of those days. I should have just stayed in bed. I couldn't wake up. My head was fuzzy.

I slept soundly, but I just didn't feel well. I didn't want to shower. I didn't want to shave. I had to work at putting on my clothes.

I had been especially apprehensive about my third chemo treatment. I didn't know why. I should have felt upbeat, considering how well the second treatment had gone. I worried whether I would react to the drugs like I did for the first treatment or like I did for the second treatment.

My anxiety may have had something to do with Becky's mom, Mary, who died after her second chemo treatment. My mind told me my situation was different, but the timing of Mary's death and the circumstances lingered. I'd loved Mary like my own mother. I expect anticipating the third chemo treatment caused the funk and a bit of depression.

I didn't eat breakfast before I went for the blood test. I should have. The lab nurse asked me if I had drunk plenty of liquids. I had not. My test showed below normal readings for my white and red blood cell counts, a first during my treatment.

As Becky and I sat in the Cancer Care Associates waiting room, an older gentleman with a beautiful mane of white hair came in with his wife and sat down across from us. The woman told us this was her husband's first chemotherapy visit. He chose not to do the buzz haircut before he came.

Becky and I couldn't help but feel sorry for him because he was probably going to lose the do and for his wife because she was going to be tracking him with the vacuum sweeper.

Only one survivor sat in the treatment unit receiving his drugs when we entered. The first two times, the room had serviced six to eight patients.

The day progressed as it had begun—not well. The nurse couldn't find a vein in my left forearm for the IV. She pricked me in one place and then lost the vein. She taped a cotton swab over that puncture and started rubbing my arm, looking for another vein. She called a second nurse to take over. This one found a vein and started the drip of Cytoxan, saline, and nausea medicine. Finding the vein took about fifteen minutes, so I was already behind schedule. I didn't feel like drinking liquids. No Cokes or hot chocolate for me.

I became antsy and wanted the treatment completed. Sitting for two hours pained my butt. The room had reading material, but reading didn't interest me.

It was always cold in that room. I had to have a blanket. The nurse said they kept the room cold because when it was too warm, patients began to throw up. Yuck, I thought. Keep it cold. I would use a blanket.

The lousy day was an omen. I expected the same euphoric reaction after the third treatment that I'd experienced after the second. It wasn't the same, though, and it crushed me. The peaks and valleys of chemo depressed me. I couldn't predict how long the peaks would last. I only knew they would end, and I was going to feel bad again.

Becky and I had planned to take our favorite vacation trip back to the hills and serenity of Branson between the third and fourth chemo treatments, between my spring semester ending and the summer term beginning. Perfect timing, I thought.

Fortunately, we'd made a two-and-a-half-hour trip to Muskogee a couple of weeks before the vacation. As we drove into town, fatigue hit me hard, totally surprising me. I had made that excursion a hundred times, round-trip the same day, and it never bothered me.

This time was different. I had zero energy. I became disoriented when we arrived. I got lost two blocks from where we had lived for ten years. I couldn't remember the names of streets or where to turn. I couldn't remember people's names and kept getting them mixed up.

Becky's two sisters who lived in Muskogee had relatively new love interests, and I couldn't remember the names of which man went with which sister. Francie had just married Steve. I finally got his name clear in my mind. But Gigi's man I couldn't keep straight. I kept asking Becky his name. I finally resorted to comparative logic. I used the Three Stooges: Curley, Moe, and Larry. I knew his name wasn't Curley or Moe. That left

Larry, and Larry it was. I remembered his name the rest of the day.

I had to take a nap and rest that afternoon. I had never had to take naps in my life.

Depression crept in. I had looked forward to our vacation and going back to Branson. The realization that I couldn't handle the trip, even for a couple of days, disappointed me and stole some of my spirit.

The further I journeyed into treatment, the easier I tired. My energy failed to bounce back as quickly as it once had, frustrating and irritating me.

When I looked in the mirror, I saw an old man. My thoughts dwelled on winter, the final season, something that had never happened before. I began to think of myself differently. I commented on my old age occasionally in conversation, as if I had already resigned myself to a life I wasn't ready to accept, a life I didn't want. My emotions welled up often. What little hair I had left on the back of my neck stood up more often. I let people get on my nerves more quickly. I scolded the dog more frequently.

Then I would wake up, hear the mockingbird singing on the rooftop, and soak up the dawn light streaming through the plantation shutters. Everything was going to be all right.

12

THE RELAY AND MY SUPPORT TEAM

I suspected something was up.

Steph and Chap surprised me in late April by showing up on our doorstep. They said we were going out to dinner on Campus Corner. Earlier in the week, Chris Krug, a former *Daily* editor, had called to say he would see me Friday night. He had let something slip.

When Becky stopped for a red light at Campus Corner, I saw a group of people looking like protesters milling around across the street. One carried a cardboard sign that I couldn't read from the distance. Where are the *Daily* reporters? I wondered.

As I watched, I thought I recognized people in the crowd. It was the newspaper staff, my students and co-workers.

Becky began honking the horn as we turned the corner. The students held up their sign that read "Team Jack." They cheered. They intended to walk in the American Cancer Society's Relay for Life on the North Oval of campus. More than fifty supporters wore T-shirts that read: "Cancer, Team Jack 2005, *The Oklahoma Daily*." The word "cancer" had a copy editor's delete mark drawn through it. Very clever, I thought: Delete cancer. Some of my students didn't recognize the editing mark, amusing to me in an ironic sort of way. I obviously had not taught them their editing marks.

Student Media sold more than a hundred of those T-shirts to our students, friends and alumni working at newspapers from as far away as *The Oregonian* in Portland and *USA Today* in Washington, D.C.

The program included OU head basketball coach Kelvin Sampson, a member of Coaches vs. Cancer. At each home basketball game, a public address announcer said, "Ladies and gentlemen, before we start tonight's game, Coach Sampson would like to introduce you to tonight's real winner . . ." Then, the coach introduced a cancer survivor. Sampson had lost his grandfather, three aunts, and a cousin to cancer. Then his mother was diagnosed.

We survivors stood in front of the podium as the emcee introduced us and told how long each of us had survived. The speakers told about what a fight it took to beat cancer and how hard it was for everyone who loved that person.

Stephanie pointed out later the large number of young cancer survivors. "It was truly inspirational," she said.

She told me about a young survivor's father who was standing in front of her: "As his daughter's name was called, I looked at him. He had tears running down his face. I did too when they called your name."

I took my hat off and placed it over my heart as a young woman sang "The Star-Spangled Banner." I was the only survivor with no hair, and I was the only man.

Becky and Stephanie walked with me on the first lap around the oval. They walked behind me on the second, as survivors took the lead.

Being called a cancer survivor for the first time made me feel strange. I was different. I was the victim. I was the minority. I felt self-conscious and embarrassed and valued and important all at the same time. That label, "cancer survivor," put me in a class of people with whom I would be identified for the rest of my life. The crowd cheered as we trekked around the oval, wearing our new American Cancer Society sweatshirts and our survivor sashes. I realized they were cheering, not because we had won the race, but because we had not lost it.

My spirit had needed a lift, and that night mingling with the relay participants and survivor supporters energized me. We hadn't eaten, but I didn't want to leave and walk across the street to Campus Corner. We did, though, and then we took Stephanie and Chap back to their car so they could go home. Becky and I picked up heavier coats and drove back to campus, where we soaked up a healing atmosphere until almost midnight.

The Relay for Life was just one of many instances when I knew God and I had help fighting the battle. Becky, Stephanie, Chap, and the rest of our family, our friends, my supervisors at work, my co-workers, and my students and Student Media alumni all overwhelmed me with support.

I could never repay Becky. Without her care and support, I didn't know what I would have done. I read a 2005 Pulitzer Prize–winning article in the *Los Angeles Times* about the marriage problems a woman survivor and her husband faced. Chemotherapy caused complications, resulting in her having a heart transplant. During the entire ordeal, she had to deal with an unsupportive life mate. The story made me want to take a shotgun and put the husband out of his misery.

Like mother, like daughter. I still had difficulty after twenty years comprehending the depth of love and support Stephanie had for me, and what I ever did to deserve her. She was the ultimate bonus when Becky married me. I'd never fathered a child, and I was always apprehensive about how Stephanie might accept me as her dad. She had already developed many of her life values by the time I met her. For her to let me into her life at age twelve, I thanked God.

Becky's sister, Gigi, mailed Hallmark cheer-me-up cards on four consecutive days. Garfield gave his advice on one: "I know things are tough right now, but just remember . . . Every flower that ever bloomed had to go through a whole lot of dirt to get there." The cards came at a particularly welcome time during my treatment—a small, but thoughtful, thing for Gigi to do, and such a lift for me. It didn't take much to make a difference in the spirit of a cancer survivor who was feeling down and vulnerable.

My supervisor Twila, going through her own severe health problems, was a rock for me—always supporting me, letting me know my career and my job were secure. My superiors up the chain of command in OU Student Affairs were equally supportive—a stark contrast to experiences related on cancer survivor message boards. Countless survivors testifying online had lost their jobs from profit-driven employers who fired them because they couldn't perform as well or because they had become liabilities to the company. One woman had worked thirty years for the same employer. The company fired her after she completed her chemo treatment.

Ryan Chittum, a reporter for *The Wall Street Journal* in New York and a former student of mine, dropped by the newsroom unexpectedly. He'd come back to cover the tenth anniversary of the bombing of the Alfred P. Murrah Federal Building in Oklahoma City. His story reported on the spectacular growth of the downtown area since that tragic event occurred April 19, 1995.

Ryan was working for the student newspaper at the time of the World Trade Center attack. He landed an internship with *The Wall Street Journal* primarily because of his coverage of Zacarias Moussaoui, a man thought at the time to be the twentieth hijacker in the Trade Center investigation. Moussaoui had lived on the OU campus for a while and taken flight-training lessons at a flight school at the Norman airport.

I lived vicariously through my students and the exciting and adventurous lives they led after leaving OU and *The Oklahoma Daily*.

Seth Prince, a copy editor at *The Oregonian* in Portland, called as soon as he found out about my diagnosis. He'd been the managing editor for the campus paper when he attended OU. His wife, Amy, covered education for the nearby Vancouver, Washington, newspaper. She'd been our editor. The two met in the student newsroom and eventually married. Six months out of college, Seth was the lead copy editor for the 2001 Pulitzer Prize–winning series about the Immigration and Naturalization Service's harsh treatment of immigrants. Back in Norman, some of the journalism professors lamented that they had toiled a lifetime and never got close to working on a Pulitzer Prize–winning story.

Heather Ratcliffe, a cops reporter for the *St. Louis Post-Dispatch* and a former editor of *The Oklahoma Daily*, also came to town to cover the anniversary of the bombing. She spent two days on campus speaking to our newspaper staff and students in my class.

These all-grown-up journalists had not forgotten their college roots—or their professor and mentor. Ryan and two other alumni—Cheyenne Hopkins, a Reuters reporter in Washington, D.C., and Stephen Spruiell, a graduate student at the

University of Texas in Austin—sent me a lucky bamboo plant. How thoughtful for three singles!

Our friends, Dr. Bill and Patti, held our hands for hours after the surgery. Patti camped in the pre-op room with us. Aside from the knowledge picked up from being a doctor's wife, she was a retired health care consultant. She provided a calming effect by telling us what was happening and what was about to happen. If something didn't seem right, she found a nurse or a doctor or an administrator and got to the bottom of it.

Ilene, a neighbor across the street whose husband had died a year earlier, became a support source for Becky. Slowly, Becky let Stephanie and Chap do things for her, something Becky had never done. A mother thinks it's her place to do the helping. Twice Becky asked Chap to put up window blinds because I couldn't lift anything.

Students continually asked how I was doing. They never looked strangely at my baldness. They never questioned the sign on my desk: "If you're sick, please keep your distance. My immune system is still on spring break." More frequently, they asked me about cancer, how I found the tumor, and what I felt. They never laughed when I put on my "Life Is Good" ball cap before leaving for the day. They understood.

One student said his mother lit a candle for me each Sunday at her church. She had just finished chemotherapy for breast cancer herself. Facing her own challenges, she lit a candle for me.

13
CHEMO'S LAST HURRAH

Certain side effects became more intense after the fourth chemo treatment. Dr. Durica said my body should have begun to adapt to the drugs. Much of the time, I couldn't tell that it had.

I couldn't stand crushed ice after chemo. Ever since I had to put crushed ice in my mouth while the oncology nurse administered the drugs, I hated ice. Putting crushed ice in my mouth reduced the chances of mouth sores. I started drinking juices and water without ice.

My shins became discolored and looked like a bad case of heat rash. I had to put lotion on my legs every day to slow the scaling. Even when I applied lotion, they still scaled by evening.

I couldn't stand the smell of engine fumes, household cleansers, cigarette smoke, bug spray, fertilizer, or any kind of chemicals. Going into the garage with its lawn mower and edger fumes and car smells gagged me. Occasionally, I didn't take my diuretic because I didn't want any more chemicals in my body.

I was irritable. I couldn't go down the street without getting upset with some driver. I had tremendous mood swings.

Norman had cottonwood trees, God's cruel joke on people with allergies. The wind made the cottony-coated seeds look like a snowstorm in May. Pollen sifted through the window screens of the sunroom, and it aggravated me. A neighbor across the street didn't keep up his lawn in a middle-income neighborhood, devaluing the aesthetics and the property values of everyone, and that aggravated me. The neighborhood association didn't enforce its covenants requiring him to keep up the place, and that aggravated me. The TV weather forecaster predicted rain and it didn't rain, and that aggravated me.

One minute, music sounded soothing. The next, it was just noise and I had to turn it off. It was too loud, too soft, too hip-hop, too heavy metal, too country, too pop. I worked in the yard for a while, and then I got tired and had to rest. My energy level fluctuated wildly. I couldn't tell the difference between my laziness and my fatigue. I was thirsty, but the water tasted foul and fruit juices added acid to my stomach.

I felt depressed one minute and optimistic and full of hope and energy the next. I felt stupid for saying—even thinking—certain thoughts, and the next minute I regurgitated them all over again. I didn't want to talk to people or hang around them. I always had been reclusive and shy, but this experience had made me more so. I didn't care to interact. I had to force myself to pray.

The drug buildup had taken its toll. The more treatments I had, the slower I bounced back. My muscles seemed to shrivel daily. They cramped often. Even my writing hand knotted up when I wrote at work. I questioned my will and resolve, something I hadn't done previously. I already worried that the cancer might come back someday and I would have to undergo chemotherapy again—or worse. I wondered if the cancer would come back next year, or the next, or the next.

I wanted this to be over.

My fifth chemo treatment didn't go the way I expected either. I had experienced a severe shortness of breath the week before my scheduled treatment. I climbed two flights of stairs to the third floor of Gaylord Hall and had to sit down on the top step because I didn't have enough energy left to walk down the hall.

When I would wake up in the morning, I felt like I had already put in a day's work and needed to go back to bed. I couldn't get used to the fatigue and the feeling of weakness. I would go to the grocery store and feel drained. I had to make myself get up out of a chair.

That shortness of breath concerned Dr. Durica. She examined me in her office the day chemo was scheduled and determined I should not have another treatment until I had a heart scan. She worried about damage to my heart. Great.

That scared Stephanie too. She had accompanied me that day. "Oh, my dear Lord," she said, "please don't let something be wrong with your heart."

Stephanie and I both thought chemotherapy was the only thing we needed to worry about. We were wrong. Dr. Durica delayed my chemo treatment a week until after the scan. Fortunately, my heart was okay.

I lacked motivation. I lost interest in my work and my life pursuits. I found myself glazing over and drifting away with my thoughts.

I also had a persistent cough. Dr. Durica put me on antibiotics for a week, which didn't help. I went through a bottle of Robitussin, and the cough persisted. Then she diagnosed the cough as a viral infection. The infection would have to run its course. Great.

Though it was a magnificent, sunshiny day, I couldn't breathe walking across campus. A convoy of gasoline-powered riding lawnmowers spewed fumes and kicked up dust while vast flower beds lay bare awaiting begonias or periwinkles or some other summer splendor.

The beds emitted toxins and odors of fresh fertilizer after landscapers had removed the dianthus. Shuttle buses roared up the South Oval, distributing passengers and diesel fumes at the same rate. The air looked like a green fog from one end of the oval to the other.

I felt like I needed a gas mask to walk the two blocks to the student union. I had never sensed the overwhelming air pollution like I did that day.

A late June thunderstorm set off the burglar alarm at 2 A.M., rousing Becky and me from a sound sleep. That prompted an in-house check with the .32-caliber pistol my dad had given me forty years ago. I didn't know if the gun would fire. Traipsing through the house in my underwear with pistol in hand, everything seemed secure. All the windows and doors remained locked with no sign of a bogeyman. Lightning or the sixty-five-mile-per-hour wind probably tripped the alarm. A similar false alarm had occurred two years earlier. The burglar alarm company rep said wind blowing against a north window caused loose wiring to set off the alarm that time.

With rain starting to pour outside and me searching inside, I saw two eyes watching me through the kitchen window. They peered at me with that let-me-in look. Abby stood there drenched and looking pitiful. I grabbed a coat and went outside barefoot to bring her around to the front of the house and into the garage. Humongous raindrops pelted my coat and soaked my skivvies and me. The wind blew so hard I couldn't hang onto the dog's collar and keep the coat hood over my head. Raindrops splashed off my bald head.

The dog, for all her good qualities, didn't have sense enough to stay dry by getting into her own bed, the bottom tier of a garden bench nestled in a corner adjacent to the sunroom and the house. Thunder and lightning scared her, and all she knew to do was yap, put on her pitiful face, and stare at me through the window.

The anxiety from the alarm and the soaking kept me awake after I got back into bed. It was creepy sometimes after an alarm. I thought no one got into the house, but I wasn't absolutely certain. I lay in bed, lights out, eyes wide open, watching the dimly lit bedroom doorway, wondering if a shadowy image would appear. The creaky sounds of wind blowing against the house and the darting shadows caused by the landscape floodlight filtering through the Japanese maple out front teased my imagination. I speculated on how fast I could get to the pistol, safely put away. I lay there thinking, calculating, waiting to go back to sleep.

Lightning zigzagged across a dark sky the next morning as thunder rumbled in the distance. Another wave of rain pushed through the metro. I sat in the sunroom listening to the rain pound the roof and watching the lightning, a bit of heaven on earth for me.

Sitting in the sunroom reminded me of sitting on an old-time porch, smelling the fresh rain, feeling the damp air, and watching the water ripple across the ground. When I was a kid, we had a front porch about three feet off the ground, complete with a swing fastened to the ceiling, a couple of metal chairs, and a black cocker spaniel.

I used to sit on that porch with Blackie and watch it rain when I couldn't play in the yard. I remembered taking afternoon naps on a pallet just inside the front screen door. The rain came down in sheets, running off the roof and causing little ditches that created a temporary moat around the porch.

This day, the rain began to move off to the northeast. Becky still slept in bed, and the dog snoozed in the garage. I sat alone with my thoughts and the tranquillity, listening to the final raindrops fade away.

I would have hated to give all that up in a lost battle with cancer. Sometimes, when my mood was just so, that thought crept into my mind.

Each summer, Stephanie carted exercise equipment, makeup trays, radios, chairs, clothes, shoes—anything she didn't want anymore—from Edmond to Norman. Becky and I rummaged through our closets, culling everything we hadn't used or worn for a couple of years. We lumped all the stuff together, stuck price tags on it, and stacked it on card tables. Before daybreak on a Saturday, we walked two houses down to Thirty-Sixth Street and pounded a sign into the ground: "Garage Sale Today."

Old sofas, doghouses, bedspreads, and bicycles meandered down the driveway from our garage to the street. Sometimes Stephanie's next-door neighbors brought their used merchandise too. Norman was a better garage sale town than Edmond.

I didn't last long outside. I was weak, and the temperature rose quickly. I had to go inside. Stephanie came in and sat with me. She watched me eat breakfast. It was too early for her to eat.

"I just enjoy being here next to you," she said.

Stephanie told me about a woman who had come to the sale while I was inside. Becky noted the woman wore both a pink bracelet and a yellow one: a breast cancer bracelet and a LiveStrong one.

"I'm fighting breast cancer, and winning," the woman said.

I'd nap a while and then go back outside and try to help out. Stephanie noticed me move out of Becky's cigarette smoke, the way she did. She had allergies. She asked me if the chemo still made me sensitive to the smoke.

"Yes, it does." But her question caused me to think of Becky, not myself, and I began to cry. Stephanie asked if I was crying because I didn't want Becky to go through the same thing I was going through.

"She's going to die just like her mother did," I said.

"Have you talked to her about it?"

"It's her life. She knows the risks."

I doubt Becky realized the depth of fear I had about her smoking. Perhaps she did. She was perceptive. But just as she wouldn't press her dad about Mary's death, I wouldn't press her about smoking. I knew smoking killed. She knew it killed. I knew how she had tried to quit. But I also knew Frank had smoked most of his life, and he lived to age eighty-two. He had a little bit of everything wrong with him that last year, but smoking didn't kill him.

I remembered something Becky said to me when we talked about her smoking after my diagnosis.

"If I get cancer, I'll just run another mile a day, and I'll deal with it."

I thought I would look forward to the final chemo session with relief and happiness. I did somewhat, but I began to dread the treatment a couple of days out. I couldn't explain it. I just didn't want to go. Perhaps I was thinking about the poor lab results, the heart scare, and the delay in the fifth treatment. I didn't want bad lab results and another delay, but I felt helpless to do anything about it.

The sixth treatment, originally scheduled for July 1, had to be delayed a week as a result of the fifth session's delay. Then the last treatment had to be changed again from Friday to Tuesday, a workday for me, because of scheduling problems in the chemo unit.

I was on edge over the weekend. I felt apprehensive and nervous, more so than before my first treatment. I sensed the intensified side effects that usually occurred after a treatment as if they were actually occurring—the god-awful taste, the dry mouth, the nausea, the weakness, the fatigue. My nostrils filled with the smell of dead cells in my body.

I felt better Tuesday morning. Adrenaline had probably kicked in. My appointment was at 1:30.

Stephanie, the cake decorator, had baked a cake to take to the cancer unit staff on my final visit. On top of the cake, she scrolled the words "Cancer sucks" with icing letters. On the side of the cake, she wrote "Thank you" to the doctors and staff.

As I sat in the recliner with the drip attached to my left arm, I watched the other survivors taking their treatments. I felt sad for them. I knew their journey wasn't complete. I knew that prior to each treatment they had to summon their courage and psych themselves up. I knew they had prayed for a successful outcome and an end to their chemotherapy, just as I had.

The feeling I had reminded me of a similar feeling I had in 1964 when my basic training ended at Lackland Air Force Base. During the last week of training, the rainbow squadrons—those new flights that had not been issued fatigues yet and still wore civilian clothes—were arriving. I knew what the rainbows were in for, and I was just glad my time was up.

This day, July 12, 2005, I knew about chemotherapy. I was just glad my time was up.

The hair on my head began coming back in. It was getting thicker and beginning to have some color. My whiskers popped out every day. It took about ten days after that last treatment for the bad taste to subside. I experienced the foul taste longer than after previous sessions.

I walked the dog six blocks a day, trying to get my strength and stamina back. One of the chemo nurses said it would likely take a year before I stopped experiencing the fatigue. Dr. Robert Gaston, the radiation oncologist, said that with my good health, six months was a more realistic time frame.

My feeling after the last chemo treatment was one of great relief. I prayed the cancer wouldn't recur. I ceremoniously threw away the Homemade Gourmet brown bag I had used to carry my lunch to work every day since chemo began in March. That sack, which contained my nausea medicine in addition to my lunch, constantly reminded me of chemotherapy. I bought a new black Thermos lunch pack to carry.

We celebrated by inviting my News Gathering class and the newspaper staff to our house for an end-of-summer and "no mo' chemo" party.

14

KEEPING LIFE IN PERSPECTIVE

Once chemotherapy ended, I began feeling confident and optimistic. I realized how my plight paled compared with the pain and suffering of so many cancer victims: advanced cancer eating away their bodies; throat cancer tearing away their larynx and esophagus; lung cancer stifling their breathing; colon cancer ripping their insides; brain cancer destroying their very essence; and financial ruin crushing their family's existence. I felt ashamed because I had let drugs control my mind and body and do my talking while I underwent treatment.

I read about the death and horrors of the war in Iraq, and that made my ordeal and my life seem inconsequential. A story in *The Dallas Morning News* told about a head nurse who spent a year with the 31st Combat Support Hospital in the

Green Zone in the heart of downtown Baghdad. Helicopters airlifted most of the wounded and dying to that hospital. Nearly twelve thousand soldiers had been wounded since the war began in March 2001.

Those nurses worked around the clock seven days a week. They didn't get to rest or take time to feel sorry for themselves. About two thousand nurses had been deployed to Iraq and Afghanistan.

The story focused on the head nurse's quick transition back into her job in the United States once her tour of duty ended. "Here, the clock hits 5:30 and you go home," she said. "Over there, you never go home."

It was most difficult sometimes to put my life and my troubles into perspective. I felt guilty for even acknowledging that something was wrong with me. If it weren't for my baldness, no one would have noticed.

I was alive. Many of those soldiers were not, or their wounds and experiences had left them maimed—emotionally and physically—and devastated for the rest of their lives.

A cancer survivor I met during a chemotherapy session was receiving treatment in the recliner next to me, and we talked. Cancer had spread throughout her midsection—stomach, vaginal area, liver, and colon. Her spirits seemed high. She was retired and I assumed in her late sixties or early seventies. She wore a small cap to cover her baldness and a happy face to greet strangers. She talked openly about her diagnosis and treatment. Her chemo treatments lasted four hours. I complained when mine stretched for two hours.

This woman was on her fifth chemo treatment with one to go. After that, she said, doctors would reevaluate her treatment. Radiation wasn't an option. She said her fourth treatment had killed about half the cancer cells. She hoped for the same success with her fifth treatment.

Then there was Molly, Stephanie's thirty-one-year-old friend at work. Molly was the first person Stephanie confided in when she found out my diagnosis in February. Three months later, Molly learned she had breast cancer. Molly's tumor was about one centimeter in diameter, so perhaps she caught it early enough to make treatment most successful.

Stephanie had cried on Molly's shoulder. Molly was a sympathetic listener and comforter. It was ironic how fate could turn and how cruel it could be.

A heating and air-conditioning estimator came to the house to provide an estimate for a new air conditioner coil. The temperature in April was 94 degrees, for crying out loud, and the AC went out. The man apologized for having a speech impediment and a slower walk. He apologized for his penmanship. He struggled with writing on the order form. He said a brain operation had caused his condition. He had a benign brain tumor removed. He said if he had waited five years, it would have been inoperable.

The number of people struggling with cancer—some 14 million diagnosed nationwide each year—amazed me. Until cancer caught up with me, I was comfortable in my own little world, and I never realized how this disease affected so many people around me.

I judged a journalism contest for the National Newspaper Association. I called the contest director because I thought I had a conflict of interest in judging the "Best Serious Column" opinion category.

The columnist I chose for first place wrote about the nation having its priorities mixed up. The writer said that if the United States could spend $150 billion to rebuild Iraq and $1 billion on planning to set up a manned station on the moon to explore Mars, it should be spending billions of dollars on cancer research. He asked why the United States could not spend $150 billion to eliminate a disease that every two days killed more people than died on September 11, 2001.

I told the woman in charge of the contest about my diagnosis and that she might want to have another judge look at the columns to make sure my bias hadn't clouded my judgment. The woman told me she was a six-year breast cancer survivor.

15

RADIATION

A Piece of Cake

My radiation treatments began August 8 in the Cancer Management Center at Norman Regional Hospital—four weeks after the final chemotherapy treatment. I had hoped treatments would end by Labor Day. That didn't happen.

The center didn't have the same negative effect on me that the Cancer Care Associates building had. The feeling wasn't about the structures or the way they looked or how nice they were. It was about what the Cancer Care building represented to me. I expected my radiation treatments to be much more tolerable than the chemo treatments. Radiation, in my case, seemed like a piece of cake compared with chemotherapy.

During my first appointment, radiation therapists set up treatment parameters on my chest. I took off my shirt and lay under a cranelike machine. The machine creaked and groaned, like it needed a squirt of WD-40, while the therapists adjusted the settings, pushing and tugging the sheet under me to position my body just so. Radiation would cover a six-inch-square area over what used to be my right breast.

As I lay on my back with my right arm arched over my head, pirouette-style, the therapists put what appeared to be a sack of beans under my head and shoulders. The beanbag formed a mold that therapists would use to help position my body exactly the same way for each of thirty-three upcoming radiation treatments.

Anna, one of the therapists, used a Magic Marker to mark up my chest, much like a cosmetic surgeon prepping me for a boob job. Her marks made my chest look like a wall of graffiti. As she scribbled, I asked if she was drawing any happy faces. She said she could do that. The little happy face washed off the next morning in the shower.

What didn't wash off were three permanent tattoos Anna had drawn. Therapists would use them as a guide for the radiation beams at 8:15 each morning five times a week for the next six weeks. I hoped the happy face's washing off wasn't an omen of what was to come.

I quickly learned the radiation routine. Each morning, I took off my shirt and T-shirt, situated myself on my back under the radiation machine's hovering eye, bent my knees so a prop could slide underneath them, and raised my right arm over my head to place it in the custom-made mold.

The machine bumped and jerked me as therapists moved the flatbed up and down a centimeter at a time to find the correct range. The jerky ride was reminiscent of the first time I drove a stick shift. To move me sideways, the therapists pulled the sheet underneath me and or they grabbed my torso and tugged and scooted it to one side or the other, all necessary to line up my permanent tattoos per the computer's instructions. I felt like a sack of potatoes.

"Cold hands," the therapists warned courteously each time before they grabbed hold of me.

"Cold hands, warm heart," I said.

On Tuesdays, Dr. Gaston, the radiation oncologist, inspected the right side of my chest, which had turned a reddish brown. Each week, it glowed a little brighter. Radiation caused my skin to burn, much like being out in the sun too long.

On Mondays, I had to weigh in. I suspected all doctors' scales were set at least ten pounds heavier than my scale at home. Noting that ten-pound difference during the first weigh-in, I told the therapist that my shoes had to be the cause of my weight gain. When I stepped on the scale a few Mondays later, the therapist kept pecking the gauge higher and higher. It finally balanced between 179 and 180 pounds.

"Hmmm, looks like you ate pretty well over the weekend," she said. "It's probably just the shoes."

Dr. Gaston redrew parameters on my chest for an extra dose of radiation. He took aim at a narrow six-inch strip surrounding my mastectomy scar, where the risk of recurrence was greatest. That area was scheduled for five extra treatments, a stronger dose of radiation. The doctor marked up the new area. As a result, the therapists had to reset the radiation machine to narrow the field where rays would strike.

One therapist took photographs of my exposed chest with a handheld camera. The only pictures therapists had taken before were X-rays. As I prepared to leave, and feeling good about myself, I asked her:

"You aren't going to put those photographs on the Internet, are you?"

I noticed one survivor regularly in the Cancer Management Center waiting room. He was about my height and weight, maybe heavier, probably younger, with dark, graying hair. Retired military, maybe. He always struck me as antsy. I didn't know what kind of cancer he had. We never talked. Sometimes he had his treatment before mine, and sometimes after.

On this particular day, I had finished my session and headed out the front door to my car. I flicked the remote to unlock the driver's door. I didn't notice a man standing in front of the car parked next to mine until I reached to open my door. I recognized him as the man I usually saw inside the waiting room. He nodded hello and smiled. His image struck me, a most ironic moment: he was smoking a cigarette.

The American Cancer Society estimated that 175,000 people died as a result of tobacco use in 2005. I was surprised at the number of college students who smoked—30 percent, according to the society. I saw them lighting up every day just outside the journalism building.

Not long after I saw the man smoking at the hospital, I watched two of my students smoking outside the glass entryway to Copeland Hall. I raised my right arm to show them the yellow Live-Strong bracelet I wore. I stuck my head out the door and asked if they realized how much fun it is to have cancer.

They wanted to know if I had ever smoked. I said no. They asked if Becky had quit smoking as a result of my cancer. I said no. They snuffed out their cigarettes and went inside.

Two-thirds of cancers were caused by preventable lifestyles, according to the cancer society. Most of those unhealthy behaviors were formed during the college-age years. That's why it was so important for young people to develop healthy life habits.

The day my radiation treatments ended, September 22, I asked Anna, the radiation therapist, whether the end of radiation meant I was cancer-free or just in remission. She hesitated before answering. I didn't know what that meant, whether she was just being thoughtful and selecting her words carefully, or whether it was something else. I held my breath. She said the word "remission" was not used much anymore.

"You're cancer-free," she said.

I exhaled.

I felt good that radiation was over, and I had a bad dose of cabin fever. Becky and I hadn't traveled out of town since the spring trek to Muskogee when I got lost. Prior to that, we hadn't left the metro since the fall a year before.

Before Becky quit her job at Dillard's, we regularly shopped in Allen, Texas, a suburb on the north side of Dallas, at the outlet mall and at NorthPark Center, an upscale mall near downtown Dallas. Liz Claiborne and Jones New York clothing stores beckoned Becky every change of season. Since she served as a Liz consultant, she had to wear Liz to work.

The effects of chemotherapy were diminishing. I wanted to see whether my fatigue or my stamina would win out on a day trip to Texas. I drove the three hours to Dallas—with only one pit stop. No getting lost. No disorientation. No fatigue.

We walked the Allen mall for four hours. I didn't tire any more so than I had during past trips. We skipped NorthPark, and I drove home, with a gas stop in Gainesville, Texas, the only break. I still felt fine, a little tired maybe, when we pulled into our driveway at the end of the day. Woohoo! I was back—and I didn't just mean back home.

16
WHAT HELPED

Winning my battle with cancer, to a significant extent, was mental. I had a positive attitude, a will to live, and a spirit that wouldn't let me quit. I knew that when I was feeling low and hurting, it wouldn't be easy to suck it up. I knew that when I was alone at night and dark thoughts consumed me, and I was scared, it wouldn't be easy. I knew.

During my struggle, especially during the chemo phase, I insulated myself with my thoughts. I focused on one thing: getting well. Nothing else seemed to matter. I occasionally thought about whether I was going to die, but I really didn't think I would. I frequently thought about how long the ordeal would last and the effect the cancer and the chemotherapy would have on my family and me for the rest of my life. I thought about a million things while dealing with uncertainty, anxiety, depression and pain of both the surgery and the treatment. I was vulnerable and fragile.

I knew I was expendable at work. I knew that I had to work or lose my livelihood and everything that went with it. I worried.

Like most people, I had to hold onto something—something to steady my thoughts, to give me hope, to let me know tomorrow would come, and that it would be better. I held on to my faith.

My attitude hit highs and lows. I didn't stay low very long, though. I bounced back like I always had. I looked on the bright side for the most part, because I didn't like to look on the dark side.

I coped with chemo by trial and error, talking to the doctor, and reading the literature. Continuing to work got me through chemotherapy. On many days, I didn't feel well, but the hubbub of the newsroom and classes kept my mind off chemo.

Exercising—working in the yard, for example—when I wasn't too tired energized me and made me feel better. I had to rest five to ten minutes every so often, but then I could go again. In June, I was burying thirty feet of low-power electrical wire for outdoor lighting about two inches below ground. I would bury three feet of line, then rest, then bury three more feet and have to rest again. A thirty-minute job took me all afternoon. I gave up walking during the summer. I also quit using the exercise equipment. I regretted that later. But some days I just didn't have the willpower or the energy to tackle those machines. Once I got out of the habit, it was difficult to get started again even though I knew it was good for me.

Keeping a journal was therapeutic for me. I was a journalist, so the words came easily. Writing allowed me to sequester myself with my thoughts. It occupied my mind and kept me from dwelling on negative thoughts. I wrote about my fears, and they didn't seem as bad anymore. I cried and didn't feel embarrassed. I told the computer what was happening to me. I developed a blogger's mentality.

I recorded highlights and triumphs of my treatment as well as problems and challenges. The journal also helped me remember details when I talked with my doctors.

I went with my instincts. If I woke up in the middle of the night and couldn't go back to sleep, I got up. If I felt like taking a nap in the middle of the day, I took a nap. If I felt like going to bed at 7 P.M., I did. Becky understood.

A flexible environment allowed me to adapt. I couldn't take the heat outside, so I stayed inside when I could. At work, I froze. I wore long-sleeved shirts through the summer. My job and my lifestyle allowed me to alter my surroundings when needed.

I maintained confidence in my doctors, and I rarely second-guessed them. I knew they were competent and were paying attention to my best interests. I followed their instructions, confident they would make me well.

Self-preservation kicked in. I got depressed sometimes, but that was natural. Anybody would.

If I hadn't, that wouldn't have been normal. I vowed to myself that cancer wasn't going to get me if I could help it.

I needed some time with my thoughts, some me time. It helped. Occasionally I didn't want to see anyone or talk to anyone. Sometimes I just wanted to listen to the birds sing or listen to music or listen to nothing at all.

Time became more precious to me, not so much the quantity of it but the quality of it. I was in no rush to hurry it along. I wanted to savor every moment of my life. I didn't have to go anywhere. I didn't have to be going every minute. I didn't have to have an agenda. I was comfortable at home, looking out over our backyard garden.

Good-bye, rat race.

17

THE LONG-TERM EFFECTS

Today, a year and a half after my chemotherapy treatment ended, I still worry about chemo's long-term effects. Psychological effects later in life have become an issue in cancer treatment too, because so many people are surviving and living longer. The fear of death, depression, disruption of life plans, body image and self-esteem concerns, lifestyle changes, and medical bills are emotional issues that haunt survivors.

I thought the aftereffects would have run their course by now, but I have wide mood swings, much more so than I had before chemo. I'm depressed more often. I get angry at the least little thing. Somebody can say something at work, something snide, and it gets under my skin. My mind won't let me quit thinking about it. I used to let pettiness roll off my back. Now I dwell on it, and it festers. It becomes a big thing. I know that isn't good for me.

During my treatments, Becky worried when my temper got out of hand. She said I was irritable, crotchety, impatient, and, at times, downright hateful. She said she never remembered me making her cry before chemo. She worried when I cried for no apparent reason and she couldn't stop me.

Becky worried, too, when she couldn't get me to wake up at night. I used to be a noisy sleeper, and I kept her awake. I breathed heavily and snored. Chemo stopped all that. My breathing became shallow, I stopped snoring, and I seldom moved, she said. Every so often, she had to reach over and see if I was still breathing.

I suspect the chemo affected my biorhythms cycle. The theory of biorhythms suggests that all of us have physical, emotional, and intellectual fluctuations that cycle periodically. When your physical cycle is at its peak, you feel strong and have endurance. When it's low, you don't. When your emotional cycle bottoms out, you're inclined to withdraw and be less cooperative, irritable, and negative about the things in everyday life. Some people say they improve their quality of life by following the dictates of these biorhythms. I believe my biorhythms got stuck in the low cycle.

Emotion still controls me, just as it did when I was undergoing chemotherapy. I've always been emotional (I'm a Libra, for heaven's sake), but this is a bit over the top.

I'm more reclusive. My natural shyness seems to have reasserted itself. I've always had to interact because my jobs—in retail, in newspaper management, and at the university—required it. I forced my personality to adjust to the business and professional world. I made the effort to socialize. Now that shyness, that tendency to avoid participating, has reemerged, and I can't fight it as easily as I once did. I enjoy one-on-one interaction. I thrive on it actually, but as the number of people grows in a setting, my level of withdrawal increases.

A newspaper friend of mine in Muskogee once asked if I was antisocial.

"That's an odd question," I thought, with a hint of indignation. "Of course I'm not."

Now I'm not so sure. Maybe he was right.

I fear I'm having a relapse of a childhood malady, one I made the mistake of telling my mother about after a hard day of chores. We always had milk cows on our acreage, and I liked to watch them eat. Strange, I know. As a kid, I even liked to watch my big brother, home from the Navy, eat. He loved fried chicken. (Okay, so I had a fetish.) After a particularly enjoyable session of watching our cows munch their grain for supper, I told my mother that when I grew up, I wanted to be a cow.

Dumbfounded, she asked why.

"Because all they do is eat and sleep."

My mother chastised me at some length and lectured me about ambition and initiative, drive and gumption, responsibility and get-up-and-go, and those sorts of things.

"Chemo brain" concerns me. I thought the oncology nurse was pulling my leg when she said something called chemo brain causes temporary memory loss and disorientation. "Chemo brain?" I thought. "Get out of here." I Googled "chemo brain" to see whether it existed. The Internet search engine located 766,000 relevant sites.

Chemo brain is a lesser-known side effect. People usually associate chemotherapy with pain, diarrhea, constipation, mouth sores, hair loss, nausea, and vomiting. Chemo brain is a cognitive dysfunction. As survivors try to get back into a normal routine, they may have difficulty concentrating or juggling multiple tasks. Doctors don't understand what causes it or who is likely to experience it.

Becky still worries about chemo brain. She says that during my treatments I would forget things one minute after she told me something. I had never done that. I would ask what time she was coming home from work because her schedule fluctuated. She would say 6:30. Five minutes later, I would forget what she said. I would ask again, "What time do you get off work?"

We would leave the house to go to Sam's, the discount club. At the intersection to leave the neighborhood, I would turn the wrong way.

"Where're you going?" Becky would ask.

"To Wal-Mart."

"We're not going to Wal-Mart. We're going to Sam's," she would snap.

She found it annoying—and scary.

"Did I take my medicine?"

"Yes, you did."

Fifteen minutes later: "Have I taken my medication today?"

"Yes, I told you. You already took it."

My lapses in short-term memory bother me too. I don't know if it's old age creeping up, lack of concentration, chemo aftereffects, or a combination of them. Since I didn't notice it before chemo, I suspect the condition has something to do with the poison and what it did to my brain cells. Researchers are finding that chemotherapy drugs used to treat cancer can damage the brain and that the effect can linger years after treatment.

Last summer, I bumped into the vice president for Student Affairs, one of my superiors, buying begonias at Home Depot. I knew him well. I called him by name when I greeted him. Five minutes later, I couldn't remember his name.

In December, a couple of months ago, I forgot Becky's birthday. I had never forgotten before. That night, Stephanie called to wish her mother a happy birthday. I was eavesdropping in my favorite chair next to Becky.

"No, he didn't," she said in a quiet voice.

At that instant, I remembered.

"It's your birthday today!" I interrupted. "Today's your birthday, isn't it? Why didn't you remind me? Why didn't you say something?"

"I thought you were just waiting until tonight to surprise me. You've done that before."

My heart sank, and I became extremely angry with myself. I pouted the rest of the evening, disappointing her even more, I'm sure. I hated that I had forgotten. Some husbands may not care about their wife's birthday, but I did. I didn't know what to say to her.

At school a couple of weeks ago, I couldn't think of three different words in one conversation.

"What's the word I'm trying to think of?" I asked the student.

"Gratuitously?"

"Yes, that's it. Gratuitously."

Twice more, I couldn't think of a word. I had to restructure my sentence. The student probably thought she was talking to the proverbial absent-minded professor. I felt embarrassed.

Thoughts flit through my mind. Occasionally, I forget them almost as quickly as they pop into my head. I'll be thinking of something to say, and just before I open my mouth, I can't remember what it was. I suppose that could be a good thing, depending on what I was going to say.

"Let's talk about sex."

I remember flashing that newspaper display type on the overhead in class as an example of an attention-grabbing headline a few years ago. A husky thirty-something woman sitting on the front row fumbled her pen and papers flew as she bolted from her chair and out the door. She didn't come back until she thought we had stopped talking about headlines with the word "sex" in them.

Sex affects people differently. A lot of people believe sex is only for the young. Not so. Men and women can remain sexually active until the end of their lives.

Not to brag or anything, but anytime I've needed to get it up, I didn't need Viagra, if you know what I mean. I've always had a strong sex drive. I'm a guy, right?

In junior high, anything in a skirt—gas station pinups, Kim Novak, even a lost and tattered snapshot of the local high school American beauty—aroused me. Brigitte Bardot, the French sex kitten who broke ground with her 1956 nude movie scene in *And God Created Woman* was my ultimate sex object. BB put the pout in lips long before Angelina. She became the epitome of sex, the standard by which I measured all women. Heck, she was the sex meter for every guy on the planet.

Skirt lengths rose during the sixties, and so did the bulge in my pants. Women began baring their breasts and burning their bras. I thought equal rights meant she was well balanced. What did I know about politics?

Over the years, the culture changed, and I changed along with it in many ways. Two things, though, have remained constant in my brain since 1956: sex and the Brigitte Bardot syndrome. An attractive woman, whether or not she resembled the sex goddess, always got a rise out of me—until chemotherapy.

Chemo ground my sex drive to a halt. I ran out of gas, sputtered to a standstill, milked the monkey dry. Fifty years of lust in my heart gone. Shoot, between a lost sex drive and chemo brain, I couldn't even remember what BB looked like.

"Now you know how women feel after going through menopause," Becky said.

I don't know if my sexual feelings will return. The "desperate housewives" haven't done anything for me yet. The literature insists my manliness will rise again. I've got to believe it will. I can't imagine lying beside a beautiful woman—my partner and lover—and not desiring her sexually for the rest of my life.

Nah, that's not going to happen. I'm a guy, right?

My toenails and fingernails took a hit during chemo. It takes months for a nail to grow back. If you've ever lost one—by wearing a shoe that's too small or working in gloves too small—you know what I mean.

At school, I inadvertently scratched my fingernail across the blackboard while using the eraser. The screeching sound sent the students into shivers. My sweeping motion split the fingernail on my bird finger down the middle almost to the quick—payback, I assumed, for that finger's abundant use over the years. The split didn't particularly hurt. The fingernail was dead already. I still have to use an emery board because of hangnails. The middle of the nail keeps re-splitting before it grows out enough to use clippers.

The toenails on my big toes still haven't grown back. Both toenails died and turned an ugly black. Eventually, they fell off without my realizing it. Becky found the first one on the closet floor.

"Eek! What's that?" She picked up the odd-shaped object and examined it. She thought it was a piece of peanut brittle candy the neighbor had given us. She sniffed it.

"Eek!" She was wrong.

I often notice the tops of my shoes speckled with tiny white flecks. My Johnston & Murphy dress blacks look like they have dandruff or like I wore them to paint the house. I polish them with an Instant Shine sponge each morning, so I know the spattering isn't dust and dirt from wear. Dead skin cells sift down my pants leg, giving my shine that salt-and-pepper look. During chemo, I had begun using a dry skin lotion after showering. It's not working that well.

Women at a Breast Cancer Month discussion group asked me if having breast cancer made me feel differently about women's breasts. "I've always been a breast man," I told them. "But, yes, having breast cancer made me more sensitive to women and how they might react to having breast cancer."

The women asked if I viewed my breasts any differently. I have a six-inch surgery scar across my chest and I have no nipple on the right side. I don't sweat on that side. Other than that, I don't view my breasts any differently. Neither do I take off my undershirt when anyone is looking.

They asked if having a woman's disease bothered me.

"No, it didn't," I said. "To me, cancer is cancer."

Whether the insurance company or Medicare will balk in the future concerns me. I've got three and a half years of monitoring left. Before my treatment began, I wondered whether the insurance company would pay and agree to the treatments prescribed. My company, Aetna—through OU's employee group plan—pleasantly surprised me.

The company contacted me within hours after my hospital stay for surgery to ask how I was doing, if I needed any medical equipment or additional services, and how the hospital and doctors treated me. The company paid without question for the treatments prescribed by my doctors and agreed to the referrals my doctors made, as far as I know.

That's not the case with many insurance companies. My sister, who died of Parkinson's disease, insisted that I, as her power of attorney, continue to pay for a supplemental insurance policy to which she had subscribed for years. I paid that organization's premium every month for eight years, and the organization never paid out a dime for her medical expenses.

Every time I submitted a bill, the response was "Oh, we don't cover that" or "Blah, blah, blah, blah, blah." I requested assistance with her prescription bills—nearly $1,000 a month—and the response was a discount card in the mail. Prescriptions at every pharmacy I already shopped cost less than at the drugstores accepting the discount card.

Becky, caught between jobs without insurance, had to take out a one-year temporary plan until she qualified for my policy at OU. When Abby broke Becky's fingers, the temp insurance company refused to pay for physical therapy for the duration her doctors ordered. Consequently, she only has about 70 percent use of her left hand now. The insurance company also refused to pay to treat the chronic pain disorder that resulted from the trauma to her fingers.

After an apparent disagreement with Cancer Care Associates, my insurance company refused to pay for follow-up visits to my medical oncologist. Dr. Durica had prescribed tamoxifen for me over the next five years. She was the one who would monitor any long-term effects of the chemotherapy and keep watch for recurrence.

I feared I would have to change oncologists and travel to Oklahoma City to see a doctor approved by Aetna. I took that to mean a doctor who didn't charge the insurance company as much money, one who was going to prescribe based on the insurance company's wishes and not necessarily on what was best for me, one who was going to keep Aetna stockholders happy, and one who would not be my first choice. Fortunately, the two companies reached an agreement at the eleventh hour. I could continue seeing Dr. Durica.

Still, the insurance company frequently refuses to pay for drugs prescribed by my doctors. Aetna dictates what drugs I take if I expect insurance to pay for them. As Becky puts it, that's just not right.

18
LIFE AFTER CANCER

Cancer has made me think about things I don't often think about. I read about a cancer survivor who said he was glad he got cancer because it made him live his life to the fullest. I'm not glad I got cancer. It took a tremendous emotional, physical, and financial toll on my family and me. But it's made me appreciate my life more. It's made me appreciate the people who love me. It's made me realize what's important to me—and what's not.

This experience made me accept my mortality. I now know I could die from cancer or some other disease—and at any time. I've come to terms better with my age. I don't feel sixty-six. I don't think of myself as old until I look in the mirror, and I think, "My God, is that really me? Where has Jack gone?" I remember my dad at sixty-five. I thought he talked slowly and moved slower. I couldn't imagine ever being that old.

I enrolled for Medicare benefits. I'm not sure if that's a depressing milestone or an occasion to celebrate. I'm certainly happy to read the newspaper's obit section each morning and find that I'm not in there. The civil service worker at the Social Security office asked me if I wanted to start taking benefits the first of the year. Absolutely not, I said, still fighting the aging process. Later, I thought, "Hello." I changed my mind. Uncle Sam owes me, and it's payback time.

Like anyone with sixty-six years of baggage, I've wondered what I would do differently in my life if I could. One particular relationship comes to mind. I had purposely distanced myself from my family as Sandra fought her demons throughout the stages of schizophrenia. Eventually she couldn't stand to be around any member of my family. I had taken to heart advice from my youngest sister, Fran. "When you get married," she said, "you choose your wife over your family. That's just what a husband does." I did that. That's just what a husband does.

Sandra and I pulled further and further away from my family. As the disease took control of her and the years went by, we didn't visit my parents' home on holidays or any other day. For the first ten years of our marriage, I owned and managed a variety store, Shoppers Town, in eastern Oklahoma with my parents, a difficult business arrangement under the circumstances. As Sandra's condition progressed into the very depths of mental illness, our relationship with my mom and dad and the rest of my family deteriorated until it was almost nonexistent—at least in my mind.

I didn't want it that way, but I felt I had no choice. Besides me, Sandra had no one left—no parents, no close friends, no confidants—except her sister, and Sandra would strain that relationship during the worst of times. She withdrew and turned against everyone. If I could live those years over again, I would figure a way to remain closer to my family and still love and take care of my wife. I was young and didn't have the life experience or the sense necessary to adequately deal with the situation. I know my decisions hurt my family. I can only pray that I comforted and protected Sandra and that my family understood and forgave me. I have to believe they did.

For twenty years, I dreaded the day Sandra would withdraw and turn against me too, as psychiatrists said she would. She never did.

I've thought about whether I've done the things in my life that I wanted to or needed to—those things that I still have some control over. As a young man, I was puzzled by the last wishes of my sister's husband, Charles, before he lost his battle with cancer. He didn't want to see faraway places or travel abroad during his final six months. He chose instead to go back to his roots—the place he was born, the town where he grew up, where he went to school, where he and my sister first lived. He wanted to revisit the memories one last time. Surprising to me, I now find myself thinking about such things.

My dad lived to age ninety-two and my mom to eighty-nine. With those genes, I used to believe I would live that long too. My brothers and sisters did not. Now I don't know. I wonder how many years I have left. I know the cancer can come back and in organs more critical next time.

I decided I would retire on June 1, 2007, four months before my sixty-seventh birthday, even though I originally had planned to teach until I was seventy. I saw how quickly my health could evaporate. I've taken pride in my life's work—educating through the newspaper and through the university. It has satisfied and fulfilled me. Some people shrivel up and die once they retire. Their work was their life. It defined them, perhaps to a fault. I don't want that to happen to me.

I spent my formative years, starting before I was old enough to walk, at the family produce business. My day care was watching my mom test cream for butterfat content. By elementary school age, I was washing the cream cans for my mother and candling, or grading, eggs that farmers brought to town every Saturday to sell to my dad. I've worked ever since. I don't want to work for the company store until the day I die. I love teaching my students, but I see something else in my future.

I want to spend more time with my wife and family. All these years, we've adjusted our lives around someone else's work schedule.

I want to go to Branson on my time schedule rather than being limited by a week of vacation in May and a week in August. I want to take Becky to Gatlinburg, Tennessee, to see the Great Smoky Mountains, a place I visited thirty-five years ago where the forest grows lush and the trout tastes good. I want to see the North Woods of Michigan and Minnesota, a vast range I've never seen. I want to see the New England countryside again. I remember eating strawberry shortcake in Vermont and shooting pictures of a young hound dog, as friendly and smelly as he could be, on the outskirts of Peacham, the most photographed town in New England. I want to see the covered bridges, the white church spires, and the maple trees in October.

I want to revisit Williamsburg, Virginia, where I once touched a gravestone dated in the 1700s. I sat in an old church pew where some of our country's founding fathers sat. I want to say hi to Mickey in Orlando. I want to eat smoked king salmon atop the Space Needle in Seattle again. I want to see the gardens of Vancouver, and the Cascades, and Jackson Hole again.

I want to try my hand at writing more books and spend my days rather than my nights writing. I want to read for pleasure rather than editing newspaper articles and grading papers. I want to walk for exercise during the daylight rather than venturing out into the cold, early-morning darkness before work.

An old high school buddy and I talked recently. He and I used to play tennis back in the sixties. He retired from the federal government at age fifty-five more than ten years ago. He plays golf regularly and takes four major trips a year. I don't care to golf, but I wouldn't mind traveling and hitting a few tennis balls.

Becky landed the full-time job at Talbots, the new clothing boutique that opened three blocks from our house. I knew she hated to quit Dillard's, but the circumstances of her father's illness made that decision a no-brainer. Both of us thought God had a reason and He would take care of us. He did.

She's back in her element, outfitting women with clothes, and the stars are aligned once again.

Before cancer, it didn't take a lot to make us happy. It still doesn't. New mums for the fall garden; a gentle rain so we don't have to water; a student who performs well; a leisurely shopping trip to Allen, Texas; a quiet Sunday morning reading the paper and working the crossword puzzle.

Cancer severely tested us. Our existence became uncertain and complicated, sometimes chaotic. Before cancer, I did well to see a doctor's office once a year. During treatment, I sometimes visited a doctor's office or the hospital or the nuclear medicine unit or the cancer center five times a week.

Becky and I have become closer. Before cancer, I didn't believe that possible. After cancer, I know it is.

My relationship with God, although never in doubt, has become stronger. I'm eternally thankful that He has been merciful with me and given me strength when I needed it most—and given me life when I wanted it most.

I've never been happier than now—cancer and all. I have my Becky, who's everything I ever wanted—and more—in a life mate; I have Stephanie and Chap, who make my life complete; I have other family and friends; and I have satisfaction and purpose.

God's grace shines upon me.

EPILOGUE

I was sitting in the sunroom after a beautiful football Saturday: 75-degree weather, a brilliant sun, no humidity, no wind, and no particular worry. It was October 8, 2005, my birthday. It was a perfect day—except for the fact that OU had lost to Texas, and even that bit of trivia didn't seem as important to me that day as it had the day before.

Clumps of bright yellow mums circled the patio, flanked by mounds of pink begonias. The occasional vine of hot-pink periwinkle crept out of the dry creek bed. Balled yaupon holly and dwarf nandina bushes provided texture and a backdrop of greens. Red geraniums and blue plumbago spilled over the planters, and the autumn back-yard beckoned to the cardinal and the rosy-colored finch and a pair of blue jays. Tall phlox, their bloom almost spent, strained to offer the season a final flourish.

The chill of fall already had sent a litter of field mice scurrying to find refuge from the winter ahead.

A mockingbird lay dead in the next-door neighbor's backyard. I prayed he wasn't the one that gave me so much joy and hope with his early-morning reveille that spring. His song had brightened my darkest days. His stillness served as a solemn reminder of life's fleeting existence and the eternity that awaits us all.

As the sun faded in the western sky and shadows stretched from the treetops and dipped down to darken the backyard, a crescent moon appeared in the southwest. A single star accompanied it. I sat in awe of the night's wonder, and I gave thanks for my life.

I closed my eyes and felt God's presence.